T0209938

A Complete Guide To Moving A Loved One In A Long-Term Care Facility

Cheryl J. Wilson, M.S.

WESTBOW
PRESS®
A DIVISION OF THOMAS NELSON
& ZONDERVAN

WestBow Press books may be ordered through booksellers or by contacting:

WestBow Press
A Division of Thomas Nelson & Zondervan
1663 Liberty Drive
Bloomington, IN 47403
www.westbowpress.com
844-714-3454

Poem: I am the Caregiver – Written by Cheryl J. Wilson, M.S.

Editing by David B. Wilson

Author's Website: Advocacy4Seniors.com

ISBN: 979-8-3850-1008-0 (sc)
ISBN: 979-8-3850-1007-3 (hc)
ISBN: 979-8-3850-1006-6 (e)

Library of Congress Control Number: 2023919526

Print information available on the last page.

WestBow Press rev. date: 10/25/2023

Dedication

*This book is dedicated to my mother, **Judy Wilson**, the woman who gave me birth (she constantly reminds me of this fact!) My mom has always been by my side. As a 17-year-old, I was diagnosed with a life-changing illness that started a very long and challenging journey for our entire family, which lasted until I received divine healing at 34. During those years of uncertainty, my mother stayed by my side, advocating for me when I could not advocate for myself. She taught me to never give up on someone, even when doctors and society give up on them.*

My success as an advocate is directly related to following the same techniques she used when she advocated for me. The greatest gift she gave me is the knowledge that no individual is beyond help; we need to be willing to learn how to communicate with individuals in ways they can understand.

Cheryl J. Wilson, M.S.

Contents

Examples in the Book

Acknowledgments

There are so many individuals I would like to thank for helping me with this book. Some highlights include the following:

Carol Scott, the former Missouri State Ombudsman, Marilyn McCormick, and Susan Tonarely. These three were my right-hand advocates for many years while I worked for the St. Louis Long-Term Care Ombudsman Program. Years - and tears - of professional development later, we still maintain contact and have formed lasting friendships. They have offered their expertise as I worked to ensure that everything necessary has been covered in this book.

I would like to thank David Wilson, my brother, for helping me with the editing and getting me through publishing. I could never have done it without his help.

I am so thankful for all the families who have entrusted me with the care of their loved ones. Every resident is a unique individual and, when treated with dignity and respect, can achieve great things. My residents/clients continue teaching me new and exciting things daily.

Above all, I thank the Lord for all the knowledge He has given me and for giving me a second chance at life; I also thank Him for giving me the gift of compassion.

Purpose For Writing This Book

There are a lot of misconceptions about nursing homes. Most of the time, the media is only interested in showing the tragic events that occur in some facilities. You rarely hear about the positive side of living in a residential care, assisted living, or skilled nursing facility. There are far more good stories about how residents' lives are improved by the staff working hard to ensure they have the highest quality of life possible while they rehab or live the rest of their natural lives in the facility.

This book will help educate families on what they need to know to find a facility where the staff are fully qualified (trained) to meet the needs of their loved ones. Not all facilities can care for all residents. Considering the medical and psychological needs will be important in helping you find the facility that can best meet the specific needs of your loved one.

People often ask me to tell them what the best nursing homes are. I smile and tell them that they are asking the wrong question. Any business that works with people and long-term care communities is a business like any other, and there will be problems with people from time to time. What you want to know is, when a problem occurs, how does the facility react? Do they try and sweep the issues under the rug, or do they do a full investigation and work to find a resolution?

When problems arise in a long-term care community,

residents/families assume that the staff don't care. In my 27+ years of experience as a senior advocate, I have learned that, in most cases, this is NOT true. Most staff care about providing the best care possible for their residents. In many cases, the problem is that the staff did not receive the proper information or training, so they are unaware that what they are doing is wrong. This does not mean that all the staff are good, caring individuals. That is why any time there is an issue, it needs to be thoroughly investigated to ensure that everyone caring for our seniors has the compassion needed to best care for the residents in our long-term care facilities.

I AM A CAREGIVER

I am 30, I am 40, I am 60, I am over 80 years old,
I am a caregiver.
I am black, I am white, and I am culturally inclusive,
I am a caregiver.
I am rich, I am poor,
I am a caregiver.
I am comfortable with my role as a caregiver; I am
overwhelmed with all the roles I must play,
I am a caregiver.
My loved one can do many things for themselves;
mine are totally dependent on me,
I am a caregiver.
I am happy; I am depressed, lonely, tired, ill, and angry,
I am a caregiver.
I feel pride and satisfaction in my role, I feel
tired and defeated at the end of the day,
I am a caregiver.
I have lots of family and community support; I have no support at all,
I am a caregiver.
When you come to visit me, understand I am all these
things. Most of all, remember that one day, not so long ago,
I was not a caregiver. I was just like you. As we visit, know
that at any time, your circumstances could change, and you
could become a caregiver. So, offer me the friendship and
support we once shared because one day, I will no longer be a
caregiver, and then I can walk beside you on your journey!

Author,
Cheryl J. Wilson, M.S

Introduction

Over my 25 years as a senior advocate specializing in long-term care facilities, I have found that the biggest issue with seniors in facilities that don't thrive is that they should never have been placed there in the first place! Long-term care facilities, like any other business, specialize in different areas. Placing someone with dementia in a facility where most of the other residents don't have cognitive issues is a mistake, just like placing a younger resident in a facility where the population is mostly geriatric. Most of the time, the staff does not intentionally want to provide poor care, but if they have not been properly trained, they have no idea what they may be doing wrong and why your loved one is not thriving! Knowledge is Power, and you must know how to find the best facility to meet your loved one's needs. Families need to know how to find a facility that can best meet the needs of their loved ones.

The decision to move a loved one to a long-term care facility is a difficult and often agonizing one. Often, family members who care for loved ones feel frustrated, isolated, and guilt-ridden for wanting to have a break from caregiving. Not only can it become more and more difficult to care for your loved one, but the task of finding the right place for them can seem daunting and impossible for you.

When you move someone into a long-term care facility, you

must do your homework to ensure the home you move them to can meet their needs. If you take the time to find the right place, you can avoid many problems.

This book will walk you through finding a home to meet your loved one's needs. Don't rely on the recommendations of social workers or hospital discharge planners. You know your loved one better than anyone.

Disclaimer: I live and work in the State of Missouri, so there are times in this book when I refer to laws/regulations pertaining to Missouri. When you are looking to place someone in a long-term care facility, most of how you find the best facility is the same process regardless of the state you are in. However, some things, such as Medicaid requirements and specific state laws, may differ from state to state. I will do my best to point those out as I go. Contact your local Long-term Care Ombudsman Program for assistance if you have any questions about your state's laws or regulations. The Long-Term Care Ombudsman is the federally mandated advocates for residents in long-term care facilities, and there is no cost for their services. (TheConsumerVoice.org/ get help - This website will get you to a page where you can see a map of the State's Long-term Care Ombudsman programs.) I am not an attorney. The information in this book is not legal advice. What I am sharing is based on my 27+ years of experience working as a senior advocate specializing in long-term care and dementia care.

It's 2 a.m. The phone rings and wakes you out of a sound sleep. The person on the other end tells you that your mom has fallen and is in the emergency room. The doctors suspect she has a broken hip and will need surgery followed by rehab in a local skilled nursing facility. You panic because you have no idea how to select a skilled nursing facility or even how to start the process. Where can you go for help?

Relax; the book you are getting ready to read will walk you through the process of finding a long-term care facility for any Serino. By reading this book, you will learn how to find the best facility for your loved one and become proactive, not reactive, so you will be ready when an emergency arises.

— Chapter 1 —

How Do You Know When Your Loved One Needs Long-Term Care?

When deciding whether to move a loved one into long-term care, there are many factors to consider, mainly their safety and well-being. One of the most important factors is whether they can live alone safely. This includes assessing their ability to move around their home, use the toilet, maintain personal hygiene, bathe, dress themselves, prepare meals, walk, and navigate stairs.

It's also crucial to evaluate any signs of cognitive decline, such as dementia, which can affect memory, planning, completing familiar tasks, confusion about time and day, irrational thinking, and increased risk of falls due to visual and spatial perception issues. If your loved one has early-stage dementia, they might still be able to live safely at home with proper support. However, it's time to consider the next step if they cannot continue living safely in their home. You should also consider what measures need to be taken to ensure their safety at home, the cost of such support, and whether it's feasible. In some cases, the cost of providing care at home is so high that families must consider alternative options such as assisted living facilities (ALFs) or skilled nursing facilities (SNFs) to ensure their loved one's safety.

It is wrong for one family member to have to shoulder the burden of caring for a parent or sibling. It is common for siblings to unfairly expect one individual to be responsible for caring for their parent simply because they are unmarried, work part-time, or live closer to them. This can lead to resentment towards the parent and create a rift between siblings that may never be resolved. It is crucial that the responsibility of caring for a parent is shared among all family members. However, moving them to a long-term care community may be the most compassionate and appropriate option if this is not feasible.

Even if one child is responsible for caring for their parent, it is not reasonable for the other sibling(s) to not step in and help when they can. Not everyone is capable of being a direct caregiver. There are alternative ways for siblings to contribute to their parent's care, such as completing household tasks like grocery shopping, cleaning, laundry, or doing yard work. In addition, siblings can provide financial support to enable the primary caregiver to hire outside help for respite care. Until the parent is moved to a long-term care facility, it's important for the family to work together as a team to ensure their loved one receives adequate care and the person who is doing the caregiving is getting the breaks that they need.

Whether or not your loved one has any cognitive decline, you must assess or have a professional assessment done to determine whether they can live safely in their home. If the answer is no, move on to the next stage. Many times, the cost of keeping someone at home is so great that a family must consider moving their loved one to a residential care facility (RCF), assisted living facility (ALF), or skilled nursing home (SNF) to make sure they remain safe.

Know that there is a big difference between someone having a cognitive decline and someone making a poor decision. We all make poor decisions from time to time. Just because your loved one makes poor decisions does not mean they must be moved into a long-term care community. We all have a right to make decisions for ourselves that others may not agree with.

Example 1: Making A Poor Decision

> *Have you ever been prescribed medication by a doctor and stopped taking it because you felt better? It's common, but following your doctor's instructions to take all the medication is important. Not doing so would be considered non-compliant or a "poor decision." However, this doesn't mean you should lose your right to make healthcare decisions for yourself. Similarly, your loved ones shouldn't lose their right to live independently just because their choices differ from yours.*

You will know when it is time to place a loved one in a long-term care community. Don't let any well-meaning parent, sibling, or friend try and convince you that you are doing a great job and need to continue to keep your loved one at home. I often suggest to a child in this situation to tell their sibling(s) that they would be happy to share the care and that they need a break, so they will be sending mom or dad to live with them for a few months so they can take a much-needed break. Needless to say, the sibling(s) in question usually have all kinds of reasons why they cannot care for their parent, but they expect their sibling to continue to provide the care. That is not a realistic expectation; families must work together to share the responsibilities of caring for an aging loved one.

Chapter 2

Levels of Care

The levels of care can vary from state to state. When looking for a long-term care facility, check with the Long-term Care Ombudsman or your state's regulatory agency to get the specifics on the levels of care offered.

I will use Missouri as an example and break down the levels of care available to individuals who live in Missouri. When the decision has been made to move a loved one into long-term care, options are available depending on care needs. Below are the different types of licensed care facilities. This doesn't include independent living facilities or boarding homes, as the Department of Health & Senior Services (DHSS) does not license them (which doesn't mean they aren't great places- just not what we are covering today!) The levels of care can vary from state to state.

Levels for Missouri Long-term Care Facilities – Check the specifics for your state.

This chapter looks at the levels of care in Missouri that are "Licensed Facilities." A licensed facility must follow the laws and regulations set forth by the State and or Federal governments.

In Missouri, Boarding homes are not licensed by the State or Federal government. This means that they are not required to follow the same rules and regulations that the State and Federal facilities must follow. That does not mean that Boarding Homes are bad places. It means there is no oversight monitoring these facilities, so if a problem arises, you don't have the recourse you do in a licensed facility.

Licensed Facilities in the State of Missouri

Residential Care I & II

Residential Care Option I (RCF 1) is the first and least restrictive level. In an RCF 1, the resident is provided a bed, three meals daily, 24-hour protective oversight, and help with medications and activities. In the RCF level 1 or 2, the residents must be able to transfer themselves without any assistance. Some of the RCFs will not accept any resident who is in a wheelchair. The facility has an LPN who monitors medications and the general health of the residents. The LPN is not on-site all day, and the number of residents determines how often the LPN is at the facility.

Residential Care Facility II includes all the services in the RCF I plus supervision with diets, personal care, and supervision of health care under the care of a physician. The monthly rate for residential care facilities is typically between $2,000 to $4,000.

RCF II costs more than a comparable RCF I because more services are offered.

Assisted Living Facilities (ALF) also have two levels, ALF Option I and ALF Option II. ALFs provide many of the same services provided by RCF I. They also include help with Activities of Daily Living (ADLs) such as bathing, dressing, toileting, eating, transferring, or walking.

The monthly rate for assisted living is typically between $4,000 to $7,000 per month. Many of the newer memory care facilities that have opened in the last few years are licensed as assisted living, even though they may provide a level of care that looks closer to a skilled facility.

Pathway to Safety

For States other than Missouri, contact the local Long-Term Care Ombudsman Program in that State (*TheConsumerVoice. org/get help*) to learn the definition of the Pathway to Safety for that State.

Anyone placing a loved one into an Assisted Living Facility (ALF) must know and understand the Pathway to Safety requirements. Let's start by explaining what the Pathway to Safety is. Simply put, Pathway to Safety states that a resident in an RCF or ALF must be able to get out of the building in an emergency with minimal assistance in five minutes or less.

The Missouri State regulation (19 CSR 30 – 86.042 (28)) states:

"All residents shall be physically and mentally capable of negotiating a normal path to safety unassisted or with the use of assistive devices within five (5) minutes of being alerted of the need to evacuate the facility as defined in subsection (1)(C) of this rule. I/II."

Missouri 19 CSR 30 – 86.047 (57) – Applies to Residential &Assisted Living

"Residents suffering from short periods of incapacity due to illness, injury, or recuperation from surgery may be allowed to remain or be readmitted from a hospital if the period of incapacity does not exceed forty-five (45) days and written approval of a physician is obtained for the resident to remain in or be readmitted to the facility. II/III"

What is minimal assistance? According to Missouri Regulation (19 CSR 30 -86-047 (4 J), minimal assistance is defined as: "Minimal assistance may be the verbal intervention that staff must provide for a resident to initiate evacuating the facility."

"Minimal assistance may be the physical intervention that staff must provide, such as turning a resident in the correct direction, for a resident to initiate evacuating the facility; 4. A resident needing minimal assistance is one who is able to prepare to leave and then evacuate the facility within five (5) minutes of being alerted of the need to evacuate and requires no more than

one (1) physical intervention and no more than three (3) verbal interventions of staff to complete evacuation from the facility."

The following are examples of assistance that is considered more than minimal:

A. Assistance to traverse down stairways.

B. Assistance to open a door; and

C. Assistance in propelling a wheelchair.

Understanding the Pathway to Safety will go a long way in helping a family choose the appropriate community for a loved one. Again, this applies to Assisted Living Facilities. In Assisted Living Option 1, the resident must be able to make the pathway to safety in order to remain in the facility.

In an Assisted Living Option II, the facility can choose to accept resident(s) who cannot make the Pathway to Safety. If these facilities choose to except resident(s) who cannot negotiate the Pathway to Safety, they have to devise and implement an Individual Evacuation Plan (IEP) to implement in case of emergency. If a facility agrees to admit a resident who cannot negotiate the Pathway to Safety or if a resident is in an Assisted Living Option II and cannot make the Pathway to Safety, the price is usually higher, or if already a resident, the cost goes up.

The Assisted Living Option II is what some people refer to as the option to "Age in Place." In ALF II, a resident can remain there as their condition declines up to and including hospice services coming into the ALF II. Although the ALF

II gives residents the option to "Age in Place," there are some situations where this would not apply, and the resident would have to move to a higher level of care, which would mean an Intermediate Care Facility (ICF) or the Skilled Nursing Facility (SNF). Some of the reasons a resident would have to move are if they could not transfer on their own and would require two staff members for a transfer or a Hoyer Lift to transfer or if the resident was incontinent and needed staff assistance with their personal care. Another possible reason for a resident having to move to a higher level of care would be if there was a cognitive decline and they started wandering into other residents' rooms or were at risk of elopement (walking out of the facility). When a resident becomes an elopement risk, their safety is at risk. ALF, both options I & II do not have the level of staffing that a skilled community does.

Intermediate Care

The intermediate Care Facility (ICF) has the same license as a skilled nursing home (SNF). The difference between intermediate and skilled is that the intermediate only requires supervision from an LPN, and Medicare services are unavailable in intermediate care facilities. Intermediate care is eligible to participate in the Medicaid Program (vendor). There are not a lot of ICFs in Missouri- but there are a few.

Skilled Nursing Facilities (SNF)

Skilled nursing facilities include all services listed above in the previous long-term care facilities. Typically, this is what most people refer to as a nursing home. Also included are a Licensed Nursing Home Administrator and a Director of Nurses. Skilled facilities may choose to provide Medicare/Medicaid services. The monthly rate for a skilled nursing home can range from $5,500 to over $10,000 per month, with the lower-costing facilities likely being in rural areas.

When determining what level of care your loved one needs, there are several things to consider:

Will they need Medicaid at some point?

1. If so, try to get them in a Vendor Bed immediately. In order to apply for Medicaid in Missouri, the resident must be in a Vendor bed, a bed that is Certified for Medicaid. If you can get them in a Vendor bed when they first move in, you can apply for Medicaid whenever the resident meets the financial and medical requirements. If you need Medicaid and are not in a Vendor bed, they must be moved to the Vendor bed before you can apply for Medicaid.

2. Are they declining, or are they at risk of falling? It may be wise to place your loved one in a higher level of care so you won't have to move your loved one twice in a short period of time.

Continuing Care Retirement Community – CCRC

A Continuing Care Retirement Community (CCRC), sometimes known as a life plan community, is a retirement community where a continuum of aging care needs—from independent living, assisted living, and skilled nursing care—can all be met within the community. If you live in a CCRC in an assisted living apartment and need rehab, you can be moved to the skilled nursing home, get the rehab, and then return to assisted living.

When a senior or a person with a disability significant (age 21 and up) enough to require moving into a long-term care community is moved from one community to another, you will often see a decline in the resident's physical, cognitive, or social skills. This generally will improve over time as the resident adjusts to their new home. If the resident placed has a cognitive decline or dementia, it is wise to consider moving them sooner rather than later so that they can make the adjustment to their new home before there is any additional cognitive decline. If you wait too long to make a move, then your loved one may never be able to make the adjustment, and simple things like knowing how to get to their room may not be possible for them. As you look to move your loved one to long-term care, it is important to consider this possibility when choosing a long-term community. You should take your time and do all the necessary work to ensure the first home you move them to will be the last move they will need to make. By doing this, you can ensure that they will not be forced to move to a higher level of care as their health declines. In a crisis situation, after a hospital stay due to an event, stroke, heart attack, or fall, the hospital discharge planner may be in a hurry to move your loved one. Become the advocate your loved one needs and ensure that all the research is done to ensure the community your loved one is moved to can meet their needs.

Chapter 3

Payment Options

Payment Options for Long-Term Care

Private Pay: When a resident pays privately for services in a long-term care community, it means that they do not qualify for a Medicare stay, are not eligible for Medicaid, and do not have Veterans Benefits. If you have Long-Term Care Insurance, it may pay for all or part of your stay, depending on your policy. When someone pays privately for long-term care, it means all the cost of room and board and all nursing care is an out-of-pocket expense.

Medicare - Medicare is a national health insurance program in the United States, begun in 1965 under the Social Security Administration and is now administered by the Centers for Medicare and Medicaid Services.

Medicare is our country's health insurance program for people aged 65 or older and younger people receiving Social Security disability benefits for (2) two years. You or your spouse must have paid into Medicare for at least 40 quarters to qualify. Medicare has several parts.

Medicare Part A – Covers Inpatient care in hospitals, skilled nursing facility costs, Hospice care, and Home Health care.

There is usually no monthly premium cost for Part A as long as you or your spouse paid Medicare taxes while working for a specified period of time.

Medicare Part B – Covers services from doctors and other health care providers. Part B covers outpatient care and durable medical equipment (DME), such as walkers, wheelchairs, hospital beds, and other equipment. Part B covers many preventive services like screenings, shots, vaccines, and annual "Wellness Visits." Most individuals pay the monthly Part B premium amount.

When you have Traditional Medicare, you can get a supplemental insurance policy from a private company that helps pay your share of the costs of Original Medicare; this is known as Medicare Supplemental Insurance or Medigap coverage. When you have a Supplemental Insurance Plan, the plan generally covers the 20% of the costs that Part A does not.

Medicare Part C – Medicare Advantage Plans – These are an alternative to Original Medicare. These plans bundle Part A, Part B, and Part D. Advantage plans usually have lower out-of-pocket costs than Original Medicare. Most of the Advantage plans cover extra benefits that Original Medicare doesn't cover, like dental, vision, hearing, and Part D services, which help cover the cost of prescription drugs and many of the recommended shots or vaccines. The Advantage Plans are run by private insurance companies and follow the rules set by Medicare.

Traditional Medicare vs Advantage Plans – Which is Best for My Loved One?

I don't know the specifics of your loved one's situation, but here are some factors to consider when deciding if your loved one should be on the Traditional Medicare or Advantage Plan.

Traditional Medicare	Advantage Plans
Most providers are covered on these plans.	Tend to have limited providers in the network.
Most facilities accept Traditional Medicare Plans.	Only facilities in their network are covered. Depending on the plan, there may be very few facilities on the network.
	You need to check with the facility and see if they accept your plan and if the plan will pay the facility directly or if you have to pay the facility and then submit your claim to be reimbursed. If you must do this, call your plan to verify that the facility is in their network and that you will be reimbursed.
Can get a supplemental or Medigap plan to cover the 20% that Medicare will not pay after the 20th day.	They do not have supplemental plans that you can purchase, but depending on the individual plan may have an out-of-pocket cap that participants are required to pay.

When someone is in a skilled nursing facility, they can switch insurance plans monthly to ensure they have the best plan possible. This is considered a "special enrollment period." When a participant chooses to change their policy, it will take effect on the first day of the following month.

A Word of Caution: If an individual has been on an Advantage Plan for 20 years and then has to go into a skilled nursing home, they can always switch to Traditional Medicare, Part A. Sometimes, the Traditional Medicare Part B will not underwrite the Supplemental Plan or Medicare Part B. If this happens, things like services from doctors and other health care providers, outpatient care, durable medical equipment (DME), such as walkers, wheelchairs, hospital beds, and other equipment, preventive services like screenings, shots, vaccines, and annual "Wellness Visits" are not covered and would be out of pocket expenses.

Medicare Part D – Prescription Drug Coverage – Medicare Part D helps cover the cost of prescription drugs, recommended shots, and vaccines. These programs are run by private insurance companies that follow the rules set by Medicare. Using a Part D Plan can help lower the cost of drugs and help protect against higher prescription costs in the future. When you are on Traditional Medicare, you add a Medicare Part D program to your plan, and when you are on a Medicare Advantage Plan, the Part D program is included.

What's Covered By Medicare in
A Skilled Nursing Home

Medicare coverage in a skilled nursing home is limited to the resident's required daily skilled nursing care. Medicare does not cover non-skilled personal care if it is the only care needed. Medicare-covered services include but are not limited to:

- Semi-private room
- Meals
- Skilled nursing care
- Physical and occupational therapy
- Speech therapy
- Medical social services
- Medication
- Medical supplies and equipment used in a skilled nursing facility.
- Ambulance transportation to the nearest supplier of medical services that are unavailable at the skilled nursing facility if alternative transportation endangers the resident's health.
- Dietary counseling

Missouri Health Net (Medicaid), Check the Medicaid Guidelines Specific to Your State – federal and state governments fund Medicaid. Medicaid is a medical assistance program for low-income individuals. When a resident is in a nursing home, the Medicaid program that covers nursing homes is called Vendor Medicaid. To qualify for Vendor Medicaid, the resident must meet financial and medical requirements. To make an application to Medicaid, you must:

- Reside in a skilled nursing home in a Medicaid (Vendor) bed, which means the bed has been designated as a Medicaid bed.
- Be 65 or older or meet the standard for medical disability according to federal and state law.
- In 2023, you cannot have a countable assessment worth more than $5,301.85. Countable assets include cash, bank accounts including checking, savings, money market, vacation houses and property other than one primary residence, mutual funds, stocks, bonds, and certificates of deposit. In Missouri, 401K and IRAs are considered countable assets, and any cash surrender value of insurance policies.

  o Assets that are not countable include the primary residence, one automobile, and personal property, including clothing, furniture, custom jewelry, an irrevocable funeral plan, irrevocable trusts, or $1,500 of cash value in a life insurance policy in lieu of an irrevocable funeral plan.

  o A primary residence is generally not required to be sold. If it is owned by an applicant who is single, it will not be considered "available" at the time of application, but it will be subject to a Medicaid recovery lien upon the Medicaid recipient's death. If the applicant is married, there are ways to keep a primary residence "safe" from the Medicaid recovery lien while a spouse is still alive, but to do this, it would be wise to seek guidance from a qualified elder law attorney.

A good rule of thumb is that an asset is countable if the individual applying for Vendor Medicaid can access the asset and convert it to cash within (20) twenty days.

Word of Caution – Under state and federal law, individuals who transfer any assets, such as cash, investments, and real estate, to someone other than a spouse would incur a penalty if the transfer occurred within (5) five years of applying for Medicaid. If the transfer occurred more than (5) five years before the application for Medicaid, the transfer of assets penalty would not apply. Don't listen to anyone who tells you that you can give all your money away to your children and then apply for Medicaid. If you do this, you will incur a Transfer of Assets Penalty and will not be approved for Vendor Medicaid until that penalty is paid off. I have seen this happen before; it can be financially devastating for a family.

Exceptions for Transferring Assets – Missouri still allows

some exceptions to the rules for transferring assets to children and families. These include:

- A spouse.
- A child under 21.
- A blind or disabled child who qualifies for payments from Supplemental Security Income (SSI) or Social Security Disability (SSD).
- A child who has lived in the residence with the parent for at least (2) two years immediately before the parent becomes a long-term care resident and applies for Medicaid.
- A sibling who has ownership or "equity interest" in residence and lives there for at least (1) one year immediately before the individual becomes a long-term care resident and applies for Medicaid.

Example 2: Transferring Assets Can Lead To A Penalty

I had a client who wanted to apply for Medicaid. When they reached out to me, they shared that they had gotten some "bad advice" from a professional, and now they were being denied. Medicaid. When they went to apply, they were told that they could divide the $20,000 that was causing them to be *over-resourced with their children, and they would immediately qualify for Medicaid. The family did as they were told. Their children spent the money and then discovered that they had been denied Medicaid due to the "transfer of assets." They did not know that Missouri Medicaid has a 5-year look back for any transfer of assets. By giving the money to their children, they had disqualified them for Medicaid and received a penalty. This is a great example of why you need to become an informed consumer so you will know how the system works.*

Division of Assets for Married Couples

In 1989, the government instituted the "Division of Assets," which allows the spouse who does not become a long-term care resident, known as the community spouse, to keep all or part of the couple's assets. Contrary to popular belief, it does not necessarily allow the spouse who remains in the community to keep one-half (1/2) of the assets. The rule states that the spouse living in the community may keep (1/2) assets but not more than $148,620 (2023 amount).

The minimum spousal share for 2023 is $29,724.

They may also receive an allotment from the institutionalized spouse's monthly income to supplement their own monthly income – this is called the monthly maintenance needs allowance

(MMNA). The community spouse is entitled to a minimum of $2,465 of monthly income (counting his/her own income) and can receive up to $3,716 of monthly income if his/her income is not sufficient to meet his/her monthly maintenance needs allowance. Whether the income is sufficient is based on a calculation Medicaid uses for the community spouse's monthly housing expenses. An elder law attorney can also assist in determining the community spouse's monthly maintenance needs allowance.

One misconception with Medicaid planning is that only the institutionalized spouse's assets are considered in the spend-down calculation, which is untrue. All assets owned by both spouses, individually or jointly, are considered countable for Medicaid purposes. Additionally, adding a child's name to a bank account does not deem those assets owned by the child for a one-half or one-third interest – the asset will still be fully countable and considered to be owned by the institutionalized spouse.

You may contact the nursing home to see if they have a Medicaid specialist who could help you with the application or could contact an elder law attorney to ensure everything is done correctly so you get all you are entitled to. The attorney will charge for their services. You could also contact your State Medicaid Agency for help.

What You Need to Have When Making an Application to Medicaid

- Proof of marriage
- Proof of age – birth certificate, driver's license, passport
- Social Security cards and other health insurance cards for both the applicant and their spouse
- Deeds to all real property – including the applicant's house.
- Bank account statements
- Stock certificates
- Certificates of deposits
- Bonds – including U.S. savings bonds.
- Verification of the current cash value and death benefit for all life insurance policies
- Prepaid burial contracts and copies of their irrevocable clause/waiver
- Annuity contracts and statements
- Proof of income – award letters for Social Security, VA benefits, pensions
- Verification of the cost of any supplemental health insurance premiums for the applicant and spouse
- If the applicant is married, all of the above information must also be provided for the applicant's spouse, even if the spouse is not applying for Medicaid.

Medical Criteria for Medicaid

To qualify for Vendor Medicaid, you must also meet medical criteria. In Missouri, this is done by what is known as the 18-point criteria. (Other States may have different criteria, so check with the regulatory agency in your State.) The skilled nursing home will do this assessment. This is determined by using a form to assess the residents' level of need in (9) areas: mobility, dietary, restorative services, monitoring (cognitive), medication, behavioral, treatments and personal care, and rehabilitation. A resident will receive a score of 0, 3, 6, or 9 in each category. To qualify for the medical criteria for Medicaid, the total score must be 18 or higher. If the score is below 18, then the resident will not meet the medical eligibility for Medicaid.

Once the Application Has Been Filed

If the applicant is single, they can continue to pay for any health insurance premiums they have and keep $50 (check your state for the allowable amount) for personal use (called Personal Needs Allowance); the rest of their income will need to be turned over to the long-term care facility.

If married and there is a community spouse, the spouse can keep the amount that has been estimated as their allotment and any allotment allowed from the institutionalized spouse. They should continue paying health insurance premiums and keep

$50 from the institutionalized spouse's income for the resident's personal needs allowance. The rest of the income must be paid to the long-term care facility.

What is a Medicaid spend down?

A Medicaid spend down applies when an individual's income is too high to qualify for Medicaid. When this happens, the individual must spend their income down to meet the Medicaid limit. Once they do this, they will qualify to be on Medicaid.

Example 3: How Can I Spend Down My Resources To Qualify For Medicaid

I had a family who found out they had to spend down $50,000 before being approved for Medicaid. They had been told by the nursing home that they had to use the money to pay for the nursing home, and when the money was gone, they would qualify for Medicaid. I explained to them what they had been told was not true. When someone has to spend down resources for Medicaid, they can use that money on anything for that resident, and it does not have to go to the nursing home. One suggestion that many individuals do not think about is spending some of the money to purchase *an irrevocable burial plan. This can bring the amount down significantly. You can spend the money on dentures, glasses, clothes, medical bills, and furniture for them, like a lift chair for their room; some people will get a mini refrigerator or a new television for the room. The bottom line is anything used for the individual can be purchased and counted for the spend down. When you are buying items for the individual, always keep copies of the receipts so you can prove the money was spent on them.*

The difference between Medicare and Medicaid

Medicare is federal health insurance for anyone 65 and older and some people under 65 with certain disabilities or conditions. Medicaid (called MO HealthNet in Missouri) is a joint federal and state program that provides health coverage for some people with limited income resources. Medicaid offers benefits like nursing home care, personal care services, and assistance paying for Medicare premiums and other costs.

It is best if you are in a bed with "Dual Certification?"

This means that the bed is certified for both Medicare and Medicaid. When a bed has dual certification, a resident cannot be forced to move just for payment purposes. So, if a facility has dual certification, you will not have to move out of the unit due to going off Medicare.

Example 4: I Do Not Want To Move Mom.

I had a client who had been moved to a skilled nursing home for rehab. The resident was not able to progress with therapy to the point where they could return home. The decision was made to keep this resident at the nursing home in hopes they would, at some point, be able to transition home. The family did not want their loved one to move off the Medicare Unit because their family member trusted the staff, and there seemed to be more staff on that unit than in the general population. The family contacted me with their concern, and I was able to confirm that the bed their loved one was in had dual certification (which means it was certified for both Medicare and Medicaid.) Since the resident was in a dually certified bed, they had the option to remain in that bed on the

Medicare Unit and could not be forced to move simply because of the payment issue.

Veterans Benefits

When looking into pension veterans' benefits, it is important to understand how VA benefits are determined. In order to be eligible for any Veteran's benefits, the individual must have been a veteran who received a general discharge, which includes any discharge other than dishonorable. Next, you need to know if this individual is a wartime veteran (served during wartime) or a non-wartime veteran. A wartime veteran is any veteran who served at least 90 days of active duty, with at least one of those days during a war period. The veteran did not actually have to be engaged in the war, just on active duty during wartime. The Veteran's Administration lists dates that will count as wartime service. As of the writing of this book, those dates are:

- Mexican Border period (May 9, 1916, to April 5, 1917, for Veterans who served in Mexico, on its borders, or in adjacent waters)
- World War I (April 6, 1917, to November 11, 1918)
- World War II (December 7, 1941, to December 31, 1946)
- Korean conflict (June 27, 1950, to January 31, 1955)
- Vietnam War era (November 1, 1955, to May 7, 1975, for Veterans who served in the Republic of Vietnam during

that period. August 5, 1964, to May 7, 1975, for Veterans who served outside the Republic of Vietnam.)

- Gulf War (August 2, 1990, through a future date to be set by law or presidential proclamation)

It is important to know if the veteran is a wartime veteran because certain benefit programs are only available to wartime veterans.

You can go to many places for help with applying for benefits. For example, you could go online at www.va.gov; you can reach out to an elder law attorney for assistance or reach out to a service representative through the VA.

Long-Term Care Insurance

Individuals who paid for a long-term care policy can look into having the policy pay for part of the cost of living in a long-term care facility. This could be any level of care, but whether or not the long-term care policy will pay for the care depends on the criteria set forth by the individual policy. Most long-term care policies have a qualifying period before the plan will start paying. In most cases, the qualifying period does not include the resident's time in rehab when Medicare pays for the rehabilitation. Some long-term care policies have "pre-existing conditions that may limit coverage. Read your policy through so you will know all the benefits your loved one is entitled to.

To determine if the long-term care policy will pay for care, you must contact the company, fill out the paperwork, and schedule a representative to assess the need.

Read through your policy before reaching out to the company so you will know what your loved ones are entitled to.

Chapter 4

How to Research Long-Term Care Facilities

Nursing Home Compare Ratings - www.medicare.gov/ nursinghomecompare/search.aspx (Any nursing home that accepts federal funds can be found on this site, along with their inspection reports.)

This federal rating system. Nursing Home Compare resulted from long-term care reform efforts included in the Omnibus Budget Reconciliation Act of 1987 (OBRA '87) and subsequent quality improvement campaigns, including one called "Advancing Excellence in America's Nursing Homes" from a coalition of consumers, healthcare providers, and long-term care professionals.

The Center for Medicare and Medicaid Services (CMS) created the Nursing Home Compare Five Star Quality Rating System to help individuals, families, and caregivers easily compare nursing homes and identify areas where they may want to ask questions. Ratings are available only for long-term care communities certified to participate in Medicare and Medicaid. Because not all long-term care communities can participate in these programs, some will not have star ratings.

Nursing Home Compare ratings come from the following three data sources:

- Health Inspections – This rating reflects the three most recent comprehensive inspections and any inspection because of complaints in the last three years. This rating weighs the most recent inspection more heavily than the other inspections. (You can click on the inspection report and view the complete report.)

- Staffing – This rating reflects two measures: the number of Registered Nurse (RN) hours per resident per day and total staffing per day, including RNs, Licensed Practical Nurses (LPNs) or Licensed Vocational Nurses (LVNs), and Certified Nursing Assistants (CNA's). This information is received by the Center for Medicare & Medicaid Services (CMS) from the Payroll Based Journal for the Nurses and Certified Nurse's Aides. This Payroll Based Journal data is reported to CMS each quarter. CMS then adjusts the hours based on the needs of the residents and assigns the staffing rating from 1 to 5 stars.

- Quality Measures – This rating combines the values of nine quality measures taken from the Minimum Data Set (MDS), which long-term care communities use to collect assessment information on residents' health, physical functioning, mental status, and general well-being. Most quality measures reflect the residents' condition in the seven days before completion of the assessment. Again, the long-term care community submits this clinical data.

- Nursing Home Compare provides a star rating for each of these three sources in case some areas are more important to an individual than others. Ratings range from one to five, with a five star as the best.

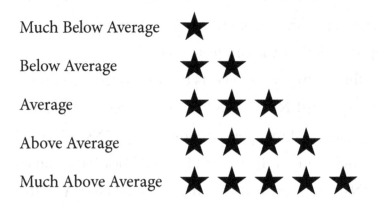

Much Below Average

Below Average

Average

Above Average

Much Above Average

A Word of Caution

When you are looking to place a loved one in a long-term care facility, don't go online and pull up inspection reports and base your decision on the results. Show Me Long-term Care and Nursing Home Compare are good starting points that can help you narrow your search, but they are only the beginning. These websites are only updated once a year when the yearly inspections are completed. A lot can happen within a facility during a year. Let's say you're looking at a facility with a 1-star rating, the lowest rating a facility can get. However, the Director of Nursing left during the year, and a new person took over. This new person came in and made many changes, and now the residents' care is excellent. However, that will not show up on these websites until after the next survey. If you never go further than what is reflected on these websites, you may miss the best opportunity for your loved one. The same is true for a 5-star facility. There may have been changes in the administration, but unless you tour the facility and see if it is a good match for your loved one, you may place them in a facility that is not as good as you thought it was.

Example 5: You Must Do Your Research

I was helping a family find a skilled nursing home for their loved one to move to. Part of the process was to go to Nursing Home Compare and get the Star Ratings for the facilities they wanted to check out. As they checked each possible home, they found two facilities with a 5-star rating. I explained the next step was to go and tour the two facilities. Once the family had completed the tour, they were surprised that what they had seen was not what had been reflected on the Medicare website. Upon investigation, I discovered that the Director of Nurses (DoN), who had been working there when the survey was done, had moved to another facility. The facility had a new DoN, and things had changed. The family then toured their second choice, felt their loved one would do well there, and went ahead with the move.

Show Me Long-Term Care - http:/health.mo.gov/safety/ showmelongtermcare/. (Any long-term care community in Missouri can be found on this site, along with their inspection reports.)

Information about all levels of long-term care communities licensed in Missouri is available at: **http:/health.mo.gov/safety/ showmelongtermcare.**

This website will access the most recent state survey results for any Missouri-licensed long-term care community, including skilled nursing, intermediate care, assisted living, and residential care. Simply select the county, city location, or five-digit zip code for the long-term care community and click "ShowMeResults."

Clicking on the inspection date or plan of correction (POC) will provide the most recent survey results, including any violations found by the Missouri Department of Health and Senior Services. If a recent inspection is not included, then the state may be in the process of completing one and adding it to the website. Individuals will also find information about any consumer complaints that the state has.

YOU KNOW YOUR LOVED ONE BETTER THAN ANYBODY, AND YOU SHOULD BE THE ONE WHO DECIDES WHICH FACILITY WOULD BE THE BEST FIT FOR THEM!

Chapter 5

Questions to Ask Prior to Admission into a Long-Term Care Facility

When considering moving a loved one into long-term care, there are several questions you should ask the facility.

Will the facility honor my loved one's durable power of attorney? If your loved one wants to withhold hydration and nutrition at the end of their life, they need to know that the facility will honor their wishes. There are facilities that will not withhold hydration and nutrition. These facilities may issue a discharge notice or send your loved one to the hospital if they choose to exercise this wish. The time to move someone is not when they are at the end of their life, so you want to address this possibility before admitting your loved one into any community.

Example 6: Make Sure The Facility Will Honor Their Advanced Directives

I had a client in a religious-based facility who started pulling out her feeding tube. Each time she pulled out the feeding tube, the facility would send her to the hospital and place it back in her stomach. The resident was not able to communicate her wishes to anyone. The facility called me to come and meet with the resident and help them determine what the next steps should be. When I met with the resident, it was clear that she could not express her wishes to me, so I asked to see her advanced directives to help me understand her wishes. As I reviewed her advanced directive, it clearly stated she did not want a feeding tube. This resident's feeding tube had been in for over two years, even though her advanced directive clearly stated that she never wanted one. On top of that, there was a handwritten note in her records where she wrote that she never wanted a feeding tube placed in her. Based on this information, I spoke with the facility administration and told them that the tube should never have been placed in her and she had a right not to have it reinserted. That's when the administrator shared with me that withholding hydration and nutrition goes against their policies. I then asked the administrator if this resident was told when she was admitted to the facility that they would not honor her power of attorney. He did not know if this had been shared with this resident. Based on his answer, I shared with them that they

could not force her to have a feeding tube and could
not discharge her because she was refusing one.

What is the restraint policy? Contrary to popular belief, it is not "against the law" for a long-term care facility to restrain a resident. The regulations that allow the use of restraints are very specific. It says that a resident can only be restrained for a medical condition with a doctor's order for a specified period of time. If a resident is restrained, very strict regulations govern the use of the restraint to protect the resident. Some nursing home facilities use restraints to treat a medical condition with a doctor's order, and others state they are restraint-free. The restraint-free facilities sometimes will say, "Our residents have a right to fall." If a facility is "restraint-free," they are still obligated to put fall precautions into place to prevent residents from falling. Some of the fall precautions may include lowering their mattress to the floor or using a personal safety device that will set off an alarm if the resident attempts to get out of their chair or bed.

The best way I know to define what constitutes a restraint is to say that anything that keeps a resident from getting up and moving freely about is considered a restraint. So, putting a resident in a bean bag chair may not be a restraint for some residents who can get up on their own but would be a restraint for another resident who cannot get up independently. Even a side rail on a resident bed can be considered a restraint if that resident has a cognitive issue and does not know how to get out of the bed on their own safely. When looking into placing your loved one in a facility, you need to understand and be comfortable with the restraint policy of the facility you choose.

How are grievances handled? If you or your loved one has a grievance, how will it be resolved? You want to know that a grievance will be fully investigated and acted upon. It is not reasonable to think that there will never be an issue. In any situation where individuals live and work together, there will be times when problems arise, which is normal. When concerns arise, ensure that the facility is committed to doing a full investigation and not blaming the problem on a resident with cognitive impairment or other medical conditions.

What is the Medicaid bedhold policy? A Bed hold is the cost a facility will charge to hold a resident's room while they are in the hospital or out on therapeutic leave. The facility usually charges the room rate per day to hold the room. So, if a facility charges $180.00 a day, then the bed hold would be $180.00 a day (even though the resident isn't in the facility at this time.) When your loved one is admitted into a long-term care facility, part of the admission paperwork is signing an agreement to pay for a bed hold. Under Federal law, you must be asked if you want to pay for a bed hold every time your loved one is admitted to the hospital. They cannot charge you if the facility fails to ask if you want to pay for the bed hold. This is often an area where facilities are sloppy about following protocol and should be monitored if your loved one enters a hospital. If you are on Medicaid and do not choose to pay the bed hold, the facility must (under federal law) put you on the top of the waitlist to be readmitted. If a facility sends you a bill for bed hold and you did not agree to pay to hold the bed, contact an advocate such as the Long-Term Care Ombudsman Program in your region to help resolve the issue.

Example 7: You Paid Bedhold

Mom fell in the skilled nursing home and was sent to the hospital. When the staff at the facility called you, they asked if you wanted to pay to hold her bed while she was in the hospital. You said "yes" so that her placement in the facility would be secured. After her surgery, she returned to the nursing home with a room waiting for her.

Example 8: You Chose Not To Pay For Bedhold

Mom fell in the skilled facility and was sent to the hospital. When the staff at the facility called you, they asked if you wanted to pay to hold her bed. You decided you did not want to pay for the bed since she was hospitalized. When it was time for her to return to the facility, there was an open vendor bed, so she was allowed to return. If all the vendor beds had been full, you would have had to place her in another facility, but her name would go up to the top of the waiting list if she wanted to return when a bed opened up.

What is the staff-to-resident ratio, and what is the turnover rate? In Missouri skilled facilities, there are no "staff ratios," The regulations say there has to be enough staff to meet the needs of the residents. In a nursing home, the number of staff required depends on the acuity level of the residents in the facility. If the acuity level increases, the number of professional staff needed to provide care can change. In assisted living facilities in Missouri, a set number of staff is required to meet the safety needs of the residents. Ask about the staff turnover rate, both administrative staff and direct caregivers. This may be a concern if the facility has a high turnover rate. Facilities with longevity with their staff are a good indicator of consistent, quality care. Some states do have a set staff ratio. When this book is being written, CMS was working on Federal Standards for staffing for nursing homes.

Are therapy services available at the facility, including physical, occupational, and speech therapy? If so, are the therapists part of the facility staff, or are they contracted out? If they are contracted out, who provides the therapy services? Sometimes, when a facility contracts out its therapy services, there can be problems if the contracted group has staffing issues and does not have the therapists to send out.

Does the facility offer special diets? These may include renal diets, low salt, ethnic diets, or diabetic diets based on the dietitian's recommendations and doctors' orders. Ask if the facility will follow your loved one's dietary needs and preferences.

Does the facility provide preventative care? This includes specialists like podiatrists, eye doctors, dentists, and audiologists.

Does the facility provide transportation to doctors' appointments when needed? Some facilities offer transportation, some insurance companies will cover the cost of transportation when necessary, and if the resident is a Medicaid recipient, the facility should arrange transportation through Medicaid non-emergency transportation.

Will the same staff care for my loved one daily, or do they change? There are advantages to having consistent staff. When a resident has the same staff member caring for them, the staff learn the routines of the residents they care for and often time will notice small changes in condition that others may not notice. Not every facility assigns staff to a regular assignment, but it is always good to know before placement.

Does the facility have a Resident Council? The Resident Council meets monthly in skilled nursing homes, and many assisted living communities also have monthly Resident Council meetings. These meetings can be run by residents or anyone the residents choose to run these meetings. The Resident Council meetings are where the residents can unite and address their concerns as a unified group. Resident Councils can also welcome new residents to the community and form different committees to meet with staff members, such as a Dietary Committee and an Activity Committee to help plan activities and outings; some resident councils will vote on an employee of the month. I have even seen some resident councils that participate in interviewing new employees. A well-run resident council is not all about complaining about issues they are not happy with; they work with the community to improve the lives of everyone living and working there.

Does the facility have a family council? A family council is a place where you can bring your concerns and expect to get some response from the facility. The facility is required to provide a space for family council and provide a staff liaison to hear and respond to concerns. The family council is also a good support group for families. Like a resident council, a family council can do fundraising to help purchase something for the residents or help the activity department increase its budget so the residents can have more opportunities. Note: Facilities are not required to have a family council. It will depend on whether the families at the facility want to be responsible for forming and maintaining a family council.

Can residents go outside to a pleasant, secure area? This is an important question to ask. Is there a patio or secure area where my loved ones can visit whenever they want to get some fresh air or visit with friends? Residents have a right to go outside, and you will want to know that there is a space available for them to do so if they choose.

Example 9: Residents Have A Right To Leave A Facility When They Choose

I received a call from a family whose father was in an assisted living facility. Their father wanted to go out on the patio to get some fresh air and was told he could not go outside without a family member or staff member with him. This particular resident had no cognitive issues and could make his own decisions. I went to the facility and discovered that residents were not allowed to leave the building unless they were with a family member or staff member. I sat down with the administration and educated them on resident rights, and from that point forward, this resident could enjoy the outdoors.

Ask for a copy of the menu and activity calendar. This will give you an idea of the meals and activities the residents have available.

Is there a "special care unit" for individuals with Alzheimer's or dementia? Suppose your loved one has early-stage dementia and will be placed in the general population.

Is there a special care unit so that if your loved one's cognitive status declines, they can be transferred to a secure unit so you will not have to transfer them to another skilled facility?

What is the wait list for Medicaid? If you are moving into a skilled facility and will need Medicaid down the road, you will want to know how long the wait is for Medicaid and how many Medicaid beds the facility has. This will give you an idea of whether or not a Medicaid bed will likely be available when you need one. If one is unavailable, you may have to move to another facility. If a facility tells you that they will have a Medicaid bed available when you need one, **DO NOT believe them**. They cannot kick someone out to make room for another resident. Most of the time, you hear this when a resident has a large amount of money, and the facility is interested in having them spend it at their facility. The bottom line is to ask to be placed in a Medicaid bed from the beginning, so this will never be a problem.

Note: Beware of facilities that tell you have to private pay for a certain period of time, for a minimum of twelve months, for example. A facility cannot contract with you to be a private pay resident for a particular time period. However, for facilities that are 100% Medicaid certified (meaning every bed in the facility is a Medicaid bed), once admitted, the facility cannot prevent you from applying for Medicaid even if they told you

at the time of admission that you would have to private pay for twelve months.

Ask to see the results of the most recent survey report. The long-term care facility is to have these results posted in an area that is easy to see. You should not have to ask; however, if you don't see the inspection report, ask where it is posted; you have a right to view the results. These survey results, also called Statement of Deficiencies (SOD), will show any deficiencies the State and the Center for Medicaid & Medicaid Services (CMS) cited in the facility. This will also show you any valid complaint investigations the State / CMS found. These are the same reports discussed in Chapter 4 that you find on Nursing Home Compare or Show Me Long Term Care in Missouri.

Be honest with the staff. Your goal is to find a facility that will best meet the needs of your loved one, and for this to happen, you need to be honest with the staff concerning the needs of your loved one. Some examples are.

A. Staff must know this before admission if your loved one is combative (fights when you try to provide care.)

B. If your loved one wanders and could walk out a door and not be able to find their way back, you must let the staff know this.

C. Let the staff know if your loved one is a "chronic complainer" and is never satisfied with anything you try to do.

D. If your loved one has a history of acting out sexually.

E. If your loved one would not accept another person sharing a room with them, let the staff know ahead of time so they can plan for them, possibly having a harder adjustment.

None of these things will automatically prevent a long-term care facility from admitting your loved one, but it will help them determine if they can meet their needs once placed. If you are not honest with them from the beginning, you will run the risk of the facility sending you a discharge letter stating that they are unable to meet the needs of your loved one. Under federal law, a facility can issue an emergency discharge notice under 30 days of admission without a reason. When I saw this happen, it was usually because the family was not honest with the facility before admission, and the facility could not evaluate the resident properly before accepting them. This is unfair to everyone, but the real victim is the resident because they must be moved to another facility.

Don't be afraid to ask questions; you need to understand everything the staff tells you. If the staff member uses terms you don't know, ask them to explain. This is the opportunity for the facility to show you why they are the best fit for your loved one. Your final question could be, "Why should I pick your facility over my other choices? Let them tell you why they are the best option for your loved one. Before leaving, get the admissions staff's name, phone number, or email so you will know whom to call with any follow-up questions. Knowing the answers to these questions will better prepare you to determine the best long-term care community for your loved one.

Example 10: Be Honest About Your Loved Ones Past

A woman complained to a long-term care community administrator, stating that she had just walked in on her husband, who was in bed with another resident. The administrator called to discuss the situation. I asked if both residents could consent and were told, "Yes." I asked if they were in a private place; they were. In this situation, there was nothing for the staff to do. Both residents were consenting adults. The administrator called me several months later and told me that the woman walked in again with her husband with this resident. When she left, she made this comment, "That's it! I've had it with this man! He's had affairs his whole life. I put him in a nursing home, and he has them there. I'm getting a divorce." I had to laugh. Why would this woman think that a man who has had affairs his whole life would suddenly stop because he is in a long-term care community? Age doesn't cause people to stop wanting intimacy.

Chapter 6

How to Tour A Facility

After doing your research, narrow your potential communities down to two or three that meet the level of care and supervision needed and any other preferred selection criteria (such as geographic location). You are ready to contact each community and set up an appointment with the staff member who oversees the admissions to inquire about touring the community and to have your questions addressed. Ask a friend or relative to accompany you on the visit. It helps to have someone who is not as emotionally invested as you are to go with you. Do not try to visit more than two or three long-term care communities in one day because they will tend to blur together.

During the initial meeting at the long-term care community, remember to discuss specific items such as costs and any extra charges for services that the basic fee does not cover. Review the long-term care community's policies, especially the restraint and bed-hold policy. Obtain a written copy of the bed-hold, which discloses any charges that residents can incur to hold their room while they are in the hospital or on therapeutic leave. When you narrow your search down to one or two facilities, ask for a copy of the admission contract to take home and review.

Tour the long-term care community with a knowledgeable staff member and observe the following:

- Is the community comfortable and homelike?
- Are there any offensive odors or smells?
- Is the temperature level comfortable?
- Do the floors and walls appear clean?
- Do residents appear well-groomed?
- Are residents "gathered" in one area?
- Are any residents "restrained"?
- Does privacy seem available to residents?
- Do residents seem comfortable around the staff?
- Do staff and residents respect one another?
- Do staff smile and engage the residents when they walk by?
- Does the staff seem energetic?
- Does staffing appear adequate?
- Does the facility provide transportation to doctor's appointments and other outings?
- Is there internet available to the residents? If so, is there an additional fee?
- What are the facility policies for hanging pictures or bringing personal items for their room?
- Does the staff respond to call lights promptly?
- Is food nutritious and appetizing?
- What are the daily activities?

- Is the activity schedule at eye level where a resident in a wheelchair could easily see what's going on?
- What is the noise level?
- How loud is the intercom system?
- How often is the intercom system used?
- Are residents who are unable to feed themselves just sitting with their meal in front of them?
- Is staff socializing more than they are working?
- Are halls crowded with equipment, soiled linen bins, housekeeping carts, etc.?
- Do residents appear engaged in "meaningful" activities?
- Is there an outdoor area where residents can go outside and visit?
- Is there a quiet area where residents can go to be alone or visit with family/friends?
- Consider talking to visitors and seeing how happy they are without staff present.
- How do they feel about the care their loved one receives?
- Do they feel the staff are attentive to the needs of their loved one?
- Sit quietly in a sitting area and observe the interactions of residents and staff.
- What are the policies for hanging pictures and bringing personal items to the room?
- If the community has a resident and family council, ask to speak with the president of the council.

Nursing homes also must post the following information daily: the total number and the actual hours worked per shift for the categories of licensed staff, unlicensed staff, registered nurses, licensed practical nurses or licensed vocational nurses, and certified nursing assistants directly responsible for resident care.

Once you have completed the facility tour, go to a quiet spot and fill out the pros/cons list (see below.) List everything on here that you learned about the facility on your visit. You should fill this out before visiting another facility to avoid confusing facilities. Once done, place it in your folder so you can pull it out and have a good recall of the visit when you are ready to decide.

After touring the long-term care community and meeting with appropriate staff, visit unannounced once or twice during regular visiting hours. Plan return visits at different times, maybe during a different shift, to observe how things operate at different times with different shifts. If the first visit was at 10 a.m., consider a return visit during mealtimes and another in the evening.

Once you have completed the tour, sit down in an area where you can quietly observe. Watch for how the staff interacts with residents, how quickly they respond to call lights or requests for help, resident-on-resident interaction, and how the direct caregivers respond to their supervisors.

See the example below of a Pros and Cons Form filled out. (Appendix 2 has a blank Pros and Cons Form.)

Name of Facility: Sunshine Valley

Address: 1111 Sun Lane

Phone Number:

Date of Visit: 05.11.2023   Time: 1 pm

Pros	Cons
The facility was clean, with no lingering smells	Halls were cluttered with equipment
There was an activity with many residents attending,	Noticed several staff members talking on their cell phones
Staff members knocked on residents' doors before entering.	Noticed the intercom system was loud and used often.

Additional Notes:

Chapter 7

What You Need to Know if Your Loved One Has Dementia?

Some long-term care facilities, skilled nursing (SNF), and assisted living (ALF) have Special or Memory Care Units. These wings are designed for residents who suffer from dementia. Dementia is an umbrella term for a group of symptoms commonly including problems with memory, thinking, problem-solving, language, and perception. The most common types of dementia are Alzheimer's, Vascular dementia, Parkinson's dementia, and Lewy Bodies Dementia. Special care units are designed to give residents suffering from dementia the specialized care they need while providing a safe, secure environment to be as self-sufficient as possible. Most of the Special Care Units are self-contained, with a private dining room and an activity room for the residents. Often, these units are more likely to have consistent staff with specialized training in working with residents suffering from dementia.

In Missouri, when you want to move a loved one to a special care unit, you can and should ask to see the community "Disclosure Statement." The Disclosure Statement defines what services are provided on the unit that makes them special or unique. This could include additional staffing, specialized training for staffing, specialized therapies, and activities that can meet the needs of residents with dementia.

How Do I Know if My Loved One Needs a Special Care Unit/Memory Care Unit?

I have been a dementia specialist for over 25 years. When I am working with a family who has a loved one with dementia, there are things I evaluate when determining if a resident needs a specialized unit.

1. Is the resident an elopement risk? If given the opportunity to walk out a door, would this resident walk out the door unsupervised? If the answer is yes, then a specialized unit would be appropriate to keep the resident safe.

2. Is the resident likely to wander in and out of other residents' rooms uninvited? If the answer is yes, placement in a specialized unit is appropriate. One of the reasons to move this resident to a specialized unit is for their own protection. Other residents may get upset when a resident comes into their room uninvited. Sometimes, when residents with dementia wander into other residents' rooms, they think the room they are in is theirs, and they may go through the drawers and may try and walk out of the room with items that don't belong

to them. Understandably, this upsets the other residents and may lead to others lashing back at the person with dementia.

3. Sometimes, residents with early-stage dementia may not be an elopement risk or wander into other residents' rooms, but being out in the general population is overstimulating for them. For these residents, being in a special care unit, which is typically smaller with more consistent staff and a regular routine, can give them a sense of more control. For these reasons, the special care unit may be an environment where these residents can thrive and have a higher quality of life.

A resident must need specialized care that is provided in a special care unit to be moved into a special care unit. Residents can't be moved to a special care unit because there's a family history of dementia, and the family wants to place their loved one in a special care unit. Under federal law, residents must be placed in the least restrictive environment. If they don't need the security of a special care unit, they should be moved to the general population. If the resident's cognitive condition declines and they would benefit from the special care unit, then a move over would be appropriate.

Families often wonder how often and when they should visit their loved one with dementia when first placed in a long-term care community. There are two schools of thought on the best course of action. First, some facilities ask that once you move your loved one, you do not visit for two to four weeks. This is so your loved one can learn to depend on the staff to meet their needs instead of the family. When the family is there every day, sometimes for most of the day, it is hard for the resident to learn to depend on the staff. This can make the transition for the resident very long and difficult. The second school of thought is to visit as often as needed and work with the facility to help your loved one adjust. Which is best? That depends on each individual. You don't want your loved one to feel like they have been abandoned by the family. However, if you work closely with the staff, they can call you if they feel that the resident needs to see you and arrange a visit. It is important for the resident, family, and staff that the resident learns to depend on the staff of the facility. As I have stated many times, you know your loved one best and will be able to determine what course of action will be the best for them.

Example 11: Resident Placed On A Secure Unit Without Cause

> *I received a call. from a Social Worker at a skilled nursing home who was working on moving a new resident into the facility. This social worker received a call from the resident's daughter, who insisted that her mother be placed in the secure unit. The*

resident did have early-stage dementia but was not an elopement risk. The daughter wanted her mom in the secure unit because she was afraid, she might try to wander away, even though this resident had never wandered away. I informed the social worker that the facility could not move a resident into a secured unit because of what may happen in the future. That would be no different than putting someone in a restraint because they might fall despite having no history of falls.

Chapter 8

How and When Should My Loved One Be Included in the Process?

The individual moving into the long-term care facility needs to be as involved in the process as they are cognitively able to be. This is going to be their home; you need their input. From the beginning of the process, ask them, "What are the most important factors to consider?" By having them involved in the process early on, they will likely be more comfortable moving in when the facility is found.

If your loved one is non-verbal due to a stroke, head injury, or cognitive impairment, it does not mean they cannot participate. Someone who is non-verbal can be asked their opinion and squeeze your hand if they agree; they can blink once for yes or twice for no. Individuals with early to mid-stage dementia have good and bad days; talk to them on a good day and get their input.

Things To Consider

- Location – close to where they now live.
  a. Are they very social?
  b. Are the facilities you're looking into close to family, friends, or their church?
  c. Do they have friends that are in a facility where they may also wish to live?
  d. Are they involved in any groups that they want to continue to attend? Veterans organizations, clubs?

- Research
  a. Once you research the facilities, sit down with your loved one and review the results.
  b. When you discuss potential concerns, let your loved one make the decision on if it would be an issue for them as a resident in the facility. Remember that this will be their home, not yours; you must let them voice their opinions.
  c. Once you have narrowed your choices down to two or three facilities, you will be ready to schedule your first meeting with the admissions staff.

- Tour your top two facilities with your loved one.
  a. Have your loved one sit down with the admissions staff and ask their questions.
  b. Tour the facility with your loved one.

c. Go during a time when they can have a meal and see if they enjoy the food. (Get a copy of the meal schedule for the month so your loved one can see what is offered.)

d. Arrange ahead of time for your loved one to meet with the Resident Council President so they can ask any questions they may have.

e. Get a copy of the activity schedule for the month for your loved one to take and review.

Example 12: When Individuals Are Involved, The Process Will Be Easier.

I had a family that needed to move their dad to a skilled nursing home. He had been living with them, but it had gotten to the point where his care was taking too much time from his daughter, and her family life was starting to have problems. The daughter thought she could find a place that she felt he would like before sharing with him that he was going to be moved. When her father found out what she was planning, he was furious and refused to enter the facility. This could have gone much differently if the daughter had sat down with her dad, explained the situation, and made him part of the process from the beginning. If she had done this, her dad may have felt like he had made the decision on what place he liked the best.

Chapter 9

Red Flags to Look For

Red Flag # 1

If your loved one will need Medicaid in the future and you will be spending their resources down in a skilled nursing home, you will want to ask the admissions person how long the wait list is for a "vendor bed." If they tell you not to worry, they will have a bed ready for your loved one when needed, and the facility is not 100% Medicaid certified; RUN, RUN, RUN! I cannot tell you how many times families have been told this, and then when they need the Medicaid bed, they are told there are none available, and they will need to move their loved one. The problem here is that each facility determines the number of Medicaid beds they have. When these beds are full, they can't kick someone out so another person can have the bed. I have had families who said that they were promised a Medicaid bed when they admitted their loved one, but when that time came, they were told they would have to move their loved one. When questioned why families are told this, they say, "We would never promise anyone a Medicaid bed." If you are looking to place someone in a facility and are told that, ask them to put that guarantee in writing or walk away. Note: I have never seen a facility put that promise in writing.

The State of Missouri updates its website annually with a list of all the licensed skilled nursing facilities, including the total number of beds and the total number of Medicaid beds. This is a great resource to use when looking for facilities, so you know beforehand whether a facility is 100% Medicaid certified and, if not, how many of their total beds are Medicaid certified. Some bigger facilities may not be 100% Medicaid certified but still have a significant number of Medicaid beds, thus increasing the chance of getting a Medicaid bed at a facility when needed. (https://dss.mo.gov/mhd/providers/pages/nfrates.htm Go to the bottom of the page and hit the Nursing Facility Rate List Excel Spreadsheet link.)

Red Flag # 2 – Beware of a Social Worker or Discharge Planner who gives you a list and tells you to select a facility.

Be an informed consumer. If you are not, you will not know that what you are being told by the hospital social worker/case manager may not be true. Often, social workers or discharge planners are pressured by the hospital administration to arrange for discharge, so they may try to pressure you into making a decision on the placement of a loved one. Too often, I have seen a hospital social worker or case managers make promises to families that either are not true or they may leave out important details.

Example 13: Discharged to a facility that could not meet his needs.

Dad fell at home and went to the hospital with a broken hip. When the time came for him to go to a skilled nursing home for rehab, the family was given a list by the social worker and told to select a facility. Dad had never been in a nursing home, and the family had no idea how to select a rehab unit. They asked the social worker for advice, and she told them that any of the facilities on the list could take their dad. The family picked a facility because it was close to their home. Almost immediately, they started receiving calls saying that Dad was refusing to go to therapy and that if he did not stop refusing, therapy would be stopped. The problem was that their Dad had early-stage dementia, and the staff at the nursing home he was moved to was not trained in how to work with residents with dementia. If Dad had been placed in a facility where the staff understood dementia, he might not have refused therapy. The problem here was that he was moved to a facility that could not meet his needs.

Examples of some "overlooked details" that can lead to a major problem for you and your loved one.

- The resident may not be old enough to qualify for Medicare, and their private insurance will not cover the cost of long-term care.

- If your loved one is on Traditional Medicare, sent to the hospital, and is admitted, you need to know if they are being admitted as an inpatient or observation status. Observation Status is paid by Medicare Part B, while inpatient status is paid by Medicare Part A. Individuals who are enrolled in Medicare Part A but not Part B will be responsible for paying the entire hospital bill if they are listed as "Observation" status.

- If someone is on Traditional Medicare but was not in the hospital for three midnights, Medicare will not pay for rehab. At the time this book is being published, Traditional Medicare requires a patient to be an inpatient of the hospital for three *midnights* before they will cover rehab in a nursing home. Oftentimes, residents are admitted to the hospital under an "Observation status" and are not considered "inpatient." The hospital is supposed to notify the patient/family within 36 hours of the patient's status, but they often do not. If a resident is transferred to a nursing home for rehab and has not been in the hospital for the three midnights, Traditional

Medicare will not pay for the rehab, and the patient will be considered private pay. The way to avoid this problem is to ask the doctor in the ER if your loved one is being admitted as an inpatient or under observation.

- Most Medicare Advantage Plans will pay for rehab based on your loved one's medical condition.

- If your loved one is on a Medicare Advantage Plan, realize many Advantage Plans have limited facilities in their network, so you need to verify that your loved one is being transferred to a nursing home in the network.

Example 14: You Need To Understand Medicare Requirements

I got a call from a family whose dad had fallen and went to a local hospital. He was admitted to the hospital, and after two days, the discharge planner called the family and told them he would be discharged to a skilled nursing home to continue his therapy. The social worker gave the family a list of several facilities to choose from with openings. The family selected a facility close to their home, and their dad was transferred the next day. The discharge planner did not know that this man had Traditional Medicare and had been admitted to the hospital under observation, not as an inpatient. Because he was not admitted as an inpatient, Medicare will not cover the cost of his rehab in a skilled nursing home. As a result, the family received a bill for the cost of their dad's rehab in the skilled facility. (Note: Even if this man had been admitted as an inpatient, he would not have qualified for rehab in the skilled nursing home because he was not there three midnights!)

Red Flag # 3 – The Doctor Ordered Long-term Care

When you are told your loved one needs to go to a long-term care facility, you must ask questions to see if you agree with what is being prescribed.

- Does my loved one need rehab in a skilled facility or long-term care? Rehab in a skilled facility is short-term, no longer than 100 days. Long-term care is for someone who's needs are too great to live in the community independently or with someone else.

- Why is long-term care needed? If the doctor is recommending long-term care and you don't understand why, ask the doctor to explain the reason for his/her recommendation.

- What are the goals for rehab?

- How long do you expect my loved one to need long-term care? Long-term care can vary in length. Someone in long-term care often will never be strong/independent enough to go home. I have seen some cases where the resident's situation has improved enough or loved ones have come forward and are able to provide a safe environment for the individual to return home.

This may or may not be an issue for you. You may know that your loved one needs to go to the nursing home for therapy so they can reach their maximum potential and return home. However, if you are surprised to hear that the doctor recommends long-term care, don't hesitate to ask questions to ensure you agree with the doctor's assessment.

Red Flag # 4 – Is There A High Turnover Rate?

If you find out that the facility has a high turnover rate, ask about the turnover rate for the administrative staff, such as administrators, directors of nurses, and social workers. When a community experiences a high turnover rate in these top positions, it can affect the quality of care that the residents receive. If the direct caregivers do not feel supported by the administration, it can oftentimes be seen in the care given to the residents.

Chapter 10

How Do I Decide?

Once you have toured, select your top two choices. Your first visit was with the admissions staff, and then you made at least one unannounced visit. You are now ready to sit down with your loved one and make your final choice. The most important person in this process is the individual being placed, provided they have the cognitive ability to decide.

Everyone who has input into the decision should be at the table. Everyone should recognize that there may be differences in opinion or disagreements, but always remember the purpose of the meeting to select the future home for your loved one that they will be most happy in. This meeting focuses on reviewing your top choices and deciding which facility is best for your loved one. Your loved one does not want to be in a meeting their loved ones are in conflict with one another.

- If they cannot participate in the decision-making process due to cognitive impairment, you need to put yourself in the shoes of your loved one. Don't base your decision on what you like the best; base your decision on what would make them the happiest. Sometimes, what is most important to you is not the highest priority for your loved one.

- Base your decision on the facts, not emotions. Just because a facility is not the prettiest doesn't mean that the care is not the best. Some of the facilities I recommend the most are not the newest facilities. At the end of the day, the most important factor is where will your loved one get the highest quality of care.

- Gather your pros & cons list from your top choices and review each one.

- As part of the discussion, ask your loved one if a pro or con is a "deal breaker" for them. If it is, remove that facility from your list.

- Make a list of any additional questions or concerns that come up so you can check it out before making the final decision.

Once all the choices have been reviewed, ask your loved one their top choice, and then you will have your answer.

Chapter 11

The Admission Process

Preadmission Screening and
Resident Review – PASRR

What is the Preadmission Screen and Resident Review (PASRR), and why is it necessary?

The PASRR is a federal requirement that ensures that all new individuals who apply for admission into a long-term care facility that accepts Medicaid (regardless of payer source) do not inappropriately place someone who does not meet the level of care criteria needed for long-term placement. Federal law states that individuals must be placed in the "least restrictive environment."

The PASRR evaluates potential residents for serious mental illness (SMI) and/or intellectual disability (ID) or related condition (RC.) A related condition, which is defined by 42 CFR 435.1010 as a disability that: a) Is attributable to i) Cerebral palsy or epilepsy; or ii) Any other condition, other than mental illness, found to be closely related to intellectual disability because it impairs intellectual functioning or would require services normally delivered to an individual with impaired intellectual functioning; b) Manifests before the age of 22, c) Is likely to continue indefinitely; and d) Results in substantial functional limitations in three or more of the following life activities: i) Self-care; ii) Understanding and use of language; iii) Learning; iv) Mobility; v) Self-direction; o vi) Capacity for independent living.

The goal is to make sure that individuals with disabilities are not institutionalized in order to receive Medicaid services that could be provided in community-based settings. If a long-term care facility is appropriate, the PASRR can provide advanced person-centered care planning by ensuring that the resident's psychological, psychiatric, and functional needs are included in the personal goals and preferences in long-term care planning.

There are two levels to the PASRR. The Level I screen is the preliminary assessment to determine if the individual might have a serious mental illness or an intellectual disability. If it is determined that the individual is positive for the Level I screen, a second in-depth Level II screen is done to determine the need, appropriate setting (long-term care vs. community setting), and recommendation for services to inform the individual's plan of care. These forms are called the DA124 A/B.

Under federal law, an individual cannot be admitted into a nursing facility unless a Level 1 screening has been completed, and if it is determined that the individual might have a mental illness or intellectual disability, then they cannot be admitted until the Level 2 evaluation has been completed and the determination is made.

If a resident comes to a long-term care facility from the

hospital, the hospital should complete the PASRR before admission. If they are coming from the community, check with the social worker from the facility you want to move them in to see what their procedure is to get this preadmission screening done.

Things to do to Prepare for the Admission Day

1. Visit the facility to see the room; this way, you will know what you can bring and where to place personal items in the room. You can ask the staff if you could set the room up with your loved ones' items before you move them in. This will allow your loved one to come into a room and see it set up with their items.

2. Ask if you can arrange lunch with the roommate before the move-in. This allows them to get to know each other and will help your loved one feel more comfortable knowing someone one day they move in. They may or may not allow this.

3. Take as many of their personal possessions as space allows. Their possessions are a connection to the past and can provide comfort when they are feeling lonely.

4. Select the clothes that you will be bringing. Remember, you have limited space for clothes, so pick the ones your loved one enjoys wearing the most. Beware of your loved ones' medical conditions when selecting clothing. For

example, If they have had a stroke, avoid bringing clothes with buttons; buttons may be difficult for them to do since the stroke.

5. Label everything! Clothes and all personal possessions, including wheelchairs, televisions, DVD players, movies, glasses, hearing aids, dentures, and anything of monetary or sentimental value, must be marked with a permanent marker.

6. Have all their insurance cards, advanced directives, living will, social security card, and powers of attorney ready to take with you. Make sure you have all the phone numbers and addresses of their doctors, family members, and anyone else you want them to be able to contact.

What to Tell Your Loved One About the Move

Ideally, your loved one was part of the process, so this will not surprise them. If the move was not something that could have been planned, such as a fall or illness, then your loved one may not feel that they need to be placed in a long-term care community and that they would be fine at home. When this happens, it adds stress to everyone involved. Here are a few suggestions, tell them:

1. The doctor recommends that you go to a nursing home that can provide more specialized care than I can give

you at home. I will visit you and be there to help you through this process.

2. I know you feel that you would be okay at home, but *I need* you to go to the nursing home so I know that you are getting the best care for yourself. I am not able to provide the care you need at this time.

3. I'm doing the best I can. I love you, but I need to take a break and care for myself and my family. I will visit you and do everything I can for you, but I need you to be in this facility now.

There is no simple way to approach this with someone who does not want to go. *Always be honest with your loved one and remain calm.* Sometimes, the person being placed will tell a child, "You promised me you would never place me in a nursing home!" I hear this often, and it is said to make the child feel guilty about putting their parent in the home. When a parent asks a child to make this promise, they are in good health. Years later, when their health declines and the children grow up and have their own lives, they expect the child to give up everything and care for them. This is not a fair request. *You did not give your parents this illness, and you are not qualified to care for them.* I would lovingly tell them you wished you could care for them, but it is impossible now.

NOTE: If a resident is competent and refuses to enter a long-term care facility, it is not legal to force them to go or sign them in against their wishes! If this happens, work with their doctor or other professionals, geriatric case manager, or elder law attorney for guidance on how to move forward.

Move In Day

Try to avoid moving in on Monday or Friday. Mondays and Fridays are the most hectic days in a long-term care facility. On Mondays, they are "recovering from the weekend, and on "Fridays" they are preparing for the weekend." The weekends are also when many of the core staff are off. I would place my loved one on a Tuesday, Wednesday, or Thursday whenever possible. This is best for the staff and ensuring my loved one has the best transition possible.

Signing the Admission Contract

This is a legal document that explains everything that is covered by the facility, as well as what is expected of you. It is a long process, and it is very important that you do not sign anything you do not understand. I recommend requesting a copy of the admission contract before the admission day so you can read it through and ensure you understand everything before signing. If you are working with an elder law attorney, ask them to review the contract and advise you on anything they feel would not be wise to agree to.

Tips when reviewing the admission contract:

1. **Responsible Party** - A nursing home cannot require anyone but the resident to be financially responsible for the nursing home expenses. If you are signing as a power of attorney, always put "POA" after the signature, indicating that you are signing as the resident's legal representative. Some facilities use the term "Responsible Party" to trick a family member into becoming financially responsible for their loved one. Typically, the term "Responsible Party" is not defined, so the family thinks they are agreeing to be the "contact person" when, in fact, the facility may be saying you are agreeing to be 100% responsible for the payment. Make sure you understand what you are signing and agreeing to. The only time you are financially responsible is if you have financial power of attorney; you are responsible for using the person's money to pay their bills. If you are the conservator/guardian or if you sign as the guarantor.

2. **Arbitration Agreement.** A certified nursing home cannot force you to sign an arbitration agreement as a condition to be admitted. In an arbitration agreement, both parties agree that any future disputes between the parties will not go to court but will be handled by a private judge called an arbitrator. The arbitration process generally is not a good idea for the resident. The process

is more expensive than a state or federal lawsuit, and the parties are responsible for paying the arbitrator by the hour. Another reason to stay away from arbitration is that arbitrators are often less sympathetic to the residents' concerns than judges or juries, and nursing homes commonly write the arbitration agreements in a way that favors the nursing home over the resident. In September 2019, CMS issued the Final Rule on Arbitration. It says that if someone signs an arbitration agreement, the facility must give them 30 days to rescind the agreement if the resident changes their mind.

3. **The 30-Day Notice** – If your loved one is private pay in a long-term care facility, most admission contracts require a 30-day notice before moving your loved one to another facility. That does not mean that you can't move them sooner, but it does mean that if you choose to move before the 30 days, the facility can charge you the difference.

If you're admitting your loved one to an assisted living, you must know that most assisted living admission contracts also have a clause stating you will give them 30 days' notice before moving mom or dad out. Next to this clause, write, "I agree to give a 30-day notice before discharge unless my loved one passes away. I will not pay for an additional 30 days if my loved one dies." This is not generally an issue with most assisted living facilities, but since 2022, I have seen this happen to several families, and even though their loved one passed away, the facility still charged the family for 30 days for not giving notice.

Once you have finished signing the admission contract, insist on a copy of the entire agreement. This is important because if you have an issue down the road, you will first want to pull out the admission contract and see what you agreed to.

Example 15: Try To Make Admission Day A Celebration

> *I had a client who was going to admit her mom into an assisted living community after her husband had passed away, and she could not live alone. Before her husband passed, the family had a home health agency providing services 12 hours a day, seven days a week. It was no longer cost-effective to have Mom live at home alone; she would need someone there 24/7. They found an assisted living close to their home that could provide the care and was affordable. Mom did not want to leave her home. The family decided to make the move as comfortable as possible. They contacted the facility and arranged for the mom, me (her case manager), and two other family members to meet the daughter at the facility on the day of the move.*

While the daughter moved Mom's things into her room and arranged them for her, the rest of us all had lunch with Mom. After lunch, we walked Mom down to her room, which was all fixed up. Mom saw her room and decided she would stay. Within a month of her Mom being at this facility, she was their best marketer, encouraging everyone she knew to move in.

Example 16: Understand The Admission Contract Before Signing!

I had a client's daughter contact me and inform me that the assisted living community where her mom had passed away sent her a bill for the full month after her death because they did not give the community a 30-notice that her mom would be leaving. After I got over the shock, I contacted the administrator and was told that the contract signed by the family stated they would give the community a 30-day notice before leaving. I shared with them that under normal circumstances, that would apply, but their mom had died. I also let her know that when a resident moves to a higher level of care, that stipulation is waived. The administrator then told me that the resident did not go to a higher level of care; she died, therefore, she is receiving no care. I was also told that the issue was non-negotiable, and the family owed them one month's rent. This is an ongoing case, and I am working with the State to close the loophole that allows the facility to do this. This is not typically how assisted living communities deal with a resident who passes away. What I now tell families when they admit a loved one into an assisted living community is to write in the contract where the 30-day notice is explained that you will pay the 30 days unless your loved one passes away. If they pass away, you do not agree to the 30-day notice and will not pay. (I don't know if this is the case in other States, but it is good for everyone to be aware of and do as a precaution.)

Chapter 12

I Care Plan

I highly recommend that the resident or family, if the resident is unable, write an I Care plan to help the community staff learn more about their loved one. This "I Care Plan" can give the staff much information about their loved ones, history, likes, dislikes, situations that cause stress, and what helps when a resident is in distress. Below is an example of an I Care Plan that a Professional Ombudsman did for her mom when she entered a long-term care community.

Nieves Fuentes Tonarely

My name is Nieves Fuentes Tonarely. I was born on August 5, 1920, and was raised in Havana, Cuba. I came from a large family with five children, Carmen, Juan, me, Maruca, and Estella. As you can see, I was a middle child and spoiled, as some say. My father ran and operated as overseer and manager of a large sugar mill. My mother stayed at home and took care of us. My father felt that girls needed to learn a skill, and cooking was not my idea of fun, so I learned to knit and crochet and played guitar.

I married my sister Maruca's husband's brother, Luis A. Tonarely. He was a tall, well-educated man in the States, a graduate of Louisiana State University. We married in Mexico, where my mother moved after my father's death. After we married, we moved back to Cuba to make our home.

Luis, my husband, was an electrical engineer and traveled with the company. I was a homemaker and virtually had no interest outside the home as women here in the States do. I loved to entertain in our home and go out with Luis. I was very close to my family. Luis and I made our home on the street behind my sister Maruca, where our backyards would join together, making one big playground for the kids as our families began.

I had one son, Luis N. Tonarely, we call him "Luisito". He was such a handful that his father decided that one was enough. That is odd, knowing that he came from a large family, larger than mine. I had always wanted a daughter. They are so pretty and fun to dress up.

Fidel Castro began his revolution and marched on our streets in Havana, claiming a better world. He would not follow through on what his claims were. My husband Luis was sent on an assignment with the company to El Salvador in South America. Luisito and I were able to travel with Luis to El Salvador. My sister Maruca and her husband called and said, "Do not come back. Things are bad. We are getting out and going to the United States. What would you like us to bring from your house?" I decided that our photos would be the most important.

Here we are, living in South America with no other family.

We were all alone in a country where we knew no one. We eventually moved to Mexico when the company dissolved after Castro took over Cuba. Many businesses had to close. Cubans were fleeing for the United States of America, and here we are in Mexico. One year later, we were able to move to the USA, where we made our home in California.

Life has been good for my family since moving to the USA. We have 8 great-grandchildren now and three grandchildren, Francesca, Ayame, and Michael. During my husband's death, Luis, on November 4, 2006, my grandson, Michael A. Tonarely, and his wife, Katrina, gave birth 13 hours later to Atticus Luis Tonarely. He has been a joy to me whenever they come to visit. I have some pictures in my room so please ask to see them.

I now live in a nursing home that my son calls an apartment. It is nice but not my home. In my home, I am used to cloth placemats, not paper or a bare table. I did not wear a bib as if I were a child. I would prefer to have it placed on my lap instead of around my neck. I didn't wear bibs at home and prefer not to start now.

If I spill, show me the way to my room and help me change into something clean.

I am used to waking up sometime between 8 and 9 in the morning. I like to have a small glass of prune juice, yogurt, a banana, and a piece of dry, dark toast. If I drink coffee, it is strong and sweet, like espresso. I do not like white bread, butter, milk, or gravies. I like baked foods, not fried. I prefer rice to potatoes; if I eat a potato, I like it dry with nothing on it. I need the roughage, so salads with vinegar and oil suit me better than having vegetables. If the veggies are in the salad, that is good; then I eat them better.

I don't drink very much liquid because I don't like to go to the bathroom and interrupt what I am doing. For me, it is an inconvenience. Chocolate is my favorite dessert; cookies are great, and chocolate ice cream makes me smile.

I like to walk for exercise or ride a stationary bike. Exercising with hand weights gives me energy. I am a stubborn woman who is used to having her own way. I do play opossum on occasion to ignore those trying to wake me or move me. I am hard of hearing, and I may not hear your request. My primary language is Spanish, and English is a secondary language. I do understand English but will go back to Spanish. Although it is now taking me longer to answer in English since I now have dementia with Alzheimer's, routing information has become more difficult and takes me much longer to respond. Please be patient with me while I search for the words to answer.

I like to do crafts such as making napkin rings, knitting and crocheting, flower arranging, painting pictures, and setting tables. I used to do a lot of entertaining with dinners and family/ friends' functions, so decorating is what I have always done. if you see me wandering in other resident's rooms and rearranging items, remember I like to decorate and not stealing their items.

I like things to look nice and home-like for a meal, not a restaurant atmosphere.

I may not remember your name daily, so remind me by introducing yourself when you see me. For example, If you see me walking down the hall, stop and say, "Hello, Nieves, this is your friend; insert your name." It doesn't matter what your job position or title is; you are my friend. All that matters is that you introduce yourself to me. It may jog a memory or help me to remember you.

When I become agitated, please put Julio Inglecia on for me. I love music and used to dance at parties and while I cleaned my home. Music is relaxing to me. I prefer Spanish Music.

Remember that I am a person, not a disease or a crazy person. I still understand what you are saying. I can't process or respond to you as I would before my memory began to fade away.

Thank you for taking the time to learn about me. I hope that this will help you care for me better and understand why I do things the way I do sometimes.

Sincerely,
Nieves F. Tonarely

As you can see, this I Care Plan gives good information to caregivers they would have never known. By doing this, the family lets staff know their mom's wishes and how to address issues that may arise. *(Thank you, Susan Tonarely, for allowing me to use your mom's I-Care Plan in my book!)*

Chapter 13

What Are My Loved One's Rights?

Long-term care facility residents have rights guaranteed and protected by law. These "resident rights" promote the principles of dignity and respect. All facilities must protect and enforce these rights for all residents.

Participate in Your Care

Residents can choose their own doctor;

Attend their care plan meeting (Skilled Nursing Homes that accept Medicare or Medicaid)

Refuse treatment: A resident can refuse any treatment, including a doctor's order. *(The most commonly refused treatment in a facility is not medication, therapy, or diet; it is bathing. Whenever a resident refuses treatment, the facility should see this as a red flag and work with the resident/doctor to find a resolution.)*

Make Choices

Residents have a right to make choices about their life that is important to them. These choices include but are limited to;

What time they get up / what time they go to bed;

What you eat / what clothes you wear;

What activities to participate in?

Be Free From Restraints

Restraints may be used when they are part of a total program to care to attain or maintain the highest possible level of well-being.

Restraints may be used, when necessary, in an emergency to protect the residents from injuring themselves or others, but they are highly regulated when they are in use.

Note: Some facilities may be "restraint-free." This is something that should have been disclosed during your meeting with the staff, so it should come as no surprise. When a facility is "restraint-free," you may have heard the staff say something like, "Our residents have a right to fall." I do not think I will ever get over a staff member telling a family that, but it does happen. Regardless of the statement, just because they are "restraint-free," the facility is still responsible for putting fall precautions into place to ensure your loved one remains safe. These can be something like lowering the bed to the floor and putting a mat on the floor so they will not get hurt if they fall out of bed.

Communicate Freely

Send and receive mail unopened;

Communicate with whomever they wish at a mutually convenient time;

Use a telephone in private;

Talk to your doctor in private.

Maintain Dignity and Respect

Be called by the name you prefer;

Have your room treated as your home/staff and visitors knock before entering,

Staff should ask permission before starting a treatment/task;

Receive medical treatment in private,

Having your personal preferences honored.

Be Fully Informed

Policies and procedures of the facility;

Access to and information concerning your personal funds;

Having information about your rights as a resident in a long-term care facility;

Current and previous state and federal inspection reports.

Voice Grievances

Voice a grievance without fear of retaliation;

Complain about any aspect of your care or living conditions;

Know the staff person responsible for grievances;

Know that the facility must respond to your complaint within three business days if the complaint is in writing. This does not mean it will be resolved in three days.

Privacy and Confidentiality

All individuals should knock on your door and wait for permission to enter;

Residents can use the bathroom in private without staff or other residents present;

Your doctor's visit, medication, and lab work should be administered in private;

Diagnosis and care needs must be kept private.

Manage Your Finances

Have access to your personal funds on weekdays during business hours;

Withdraw as much of your personal funds as you wish;

Appoint someone to handle your money;

Receive an itemized account of your bill at least every three months.

Transfer and Discharge

You can only be discharged from the facility if:

The facility cannot meet your needs;

The resident's health has improved, and they no longer need the level of care provided by the facility;

The resident is a threat to themselves or others;

The residents' bill has not been paid, or

The facility closes.

You must be given a written 30-day discharge notice and

You have a right to appeal your discharge.

Note: I highly recommend that anyone considering placing a loved one in a nursing home purchase my first book, "I Am The Resident – Becoming An Advocate For Your Loved One's Needs." This book looks at all the Federal laws that govern nursing homes and explains them in terms families can understand. There are sixty-four examples of how I used federal laws to get issues resolved when nursing homes told families things like "We are not required to do that, or Our policy is to . ."

When you move a loved one into a long-term care facility, you are their most powerful advocate. Too often, families are told facility policies, not what their loved ones' federal rights are. Knowledge is Power; I Am The Resident – Becoming An Advocate For Your Loved One's Needs will give you the tools to become the informed advocate your loved one needs.

Example 17: Residents Have A Right To A Compatible Roommate

I received a call from a social worker at a skilled facility who told me that they were having problems with two male residents who were roommates and did not get along. She said that one afternoon, while one of the residents was having lunch, his roommate moved his bed out in the middle of the hall. When the resident came back from lunch, he found his bed in the middle of the hall. The social worker wanted my help in figuring out how to handle the situation. I asked the social worker if this was a new issue, and she said, "No, these two residents have never gotten along." Once she told me this, the resolution was simple: move one of them to another room. Residents have a right to a compatible roommate. Many times, the staff can work with residents to work out issues; however, in a case like this, where the issues are ongoing, these men had a right to be placed with different roommates.

Chapter 14

What Are My Rights As A Family Member?

When a resident moves into a long-term care facility, the family should actively advocate for their loved one, ensuring the highest quality of life for them. In recent years, the focus of long-term care has changed from the medical model to a person-centered philosophy of care. This means that the resident is the primary decision maker, and what they want regarding care is the staff's primary concern. The staff must abide by their wishes as long as a resident is competent. Sometimes, family members may not agree with the wishes of their loved ones, but the staff must honor them.

With the resident's permission, family members can exercise rights that can help them advocate for their loved ones.

Initial Assessment & Care Plan Meeting – The family can participate in the resident's initial assessment in a skilled nursing home. This assessment is done within the first 14 days of a resident's admission and plays a vital role in shaping the course of the resident's care. The family member's knowledge of the resident's history, likes, and dislikes can be an invaluable information source. The home should set up a care plan meeting within seven days of the initial assessment. This is a meeting where all the department heads involved in the resident's care come together and map out a care plan for the resident. Family members have the right to attend these meetings with the resident's permission. This is a time when families can get updates on the resident's condition and voice any concerns. After the initial care plan meeting, care plans are scheduled every three months or whenever a significant change in the resident's condition occurs.

Note: Care Plans are only required for skilled facilities that accept Medicare and/or Medicaid residents. That being said, many state-only facilities (do not accept any federal funds) and assisted living communities do care plans for their residents.

Notification — Family members have a right to be notified within 24 hours of any change in a resident's condition. This includes any accident/injury, change in medical/mental status, the need to change treatment, any transfer or discharge and the reason, any room/roommate change, or any change in resident rights.

Family Councils — Family members can meet with other family members in an area provided by the facility. The staff does not have to be present, but the facility must designate a staff person who is responsible for acting on grievances and/or recommendations made by the family council.

Resident's Inventory List — This list is compiled upon the resident's admission and accounts for all their possessions.

Families have access to this to keep the list updated as they bring items in or take them home. This is particularly important to complete; it proves what your loved one brought with them when they were admitted into the facility. If something comes up missing, having this updated list is a good place to start when resolving the issue. The inventory list should include everything the resident brings into the facility of monetary or sentimental value.

Visiting — With the resident's permission, a family member has immediate and unlimited access to their loved one. Although visiting is allowed anytime a visitor does not have the right to disturb the roommate. So, if you want to visit your loved one and the roommate does not want visitors in the room, you will need to visit your loved one outside the room.

These are rights that all families have. If, for some reason, you have not been allowed to exercise your rights, talk to the staff. In most cases, a little staff education goes a long way in seeing that families get their rights honored. If you need help advocating for your loved one, contact your local Long-term Care Ombudsman Program for help. This is a free service, and they are experts in the state and federal laws governing long-term care facilities.

Chapter 15

What I Know to Be True

When speaking to community staff, always act on facts, not emotions. I know this is easier said than done. It often helps to bring a friend who does not have an emotional tie to your loved one to help when you are touring or speaking with staff.

When you are looking to move a loved one in a long-term care community, do not base your opinion on how it looks. Just because a community has a beautiful building does not mean the residents are getting quality care. In the same way, an older community is not as "pretty" but sometimes gives outstanding care to the residents. This is much like people; some of the most beautiful individuals are not the most compassionate, whereas some people I know don't have a beautiful outward appearance according to society's standard, but they have a heart of gold and are the most compassionate individuals I know. A facility can have a good inspection report and not provide warm, compassionate care to the residents. You want a facility that treats your loved one with dignity and respect so they can achieve their highest quality of life!

I often get asked, "What nursing home would you recommend I place my loved one in?" I smile and share that you are asking the wrong question. Whenever you work with people, regardless of the industry, there will be times when you experience problems. Your question should not be, "Where is the best nursing home (the one with the fewest problems.)" Your question to the staff needs to be, "When a problem arises, how do you handle the issue?" Do they sweep it under the rug with comments like "Your mom has dementia, she's just confused, or my favorite, "Since COVID, everyone is short-staffed, we are doing the best we can!" You want to move your loved one to a facility that investigates each complaint thoroughly and does not start the investigation with any preconceived ideas.

We all struggle to have control of our lives. Seniors are no different. When looking to move a loved one in a long-term care community, give your loved one as much control of the decision as they can manage. Make them part of the process. Take them on the tour, allow them to ask questions, and give their input. After all, at the end of the day, you will go home, the staff will go home, and your loved one will not; this new facility will be their home.

Do not get caught up in media stories about a facility. The media typically only reports on a long-term care facility in the midst of a tragedy. You do not hear every side of the incident; you normally only hear the negative and rarely hear the final report. Know that what they are reporting is what they were told by the person filing the complaint. Just because you hear something negative, do not assume that what you hear is the final result. If the long-term care facility meets your other criteria, go and do the research and tour just as you would in any other facility. Many good things happen in long-term care facilities that no one ever hears about.

Be careful basing your decision on what others tell you about a long-term care facility. Each family and placement is unique. Just because a friend had a bad experience with a facility does not mean you should cross that facility off your list and not do the research. Remember, the person who shared their experience with you only tells you one side of the story, their side according to what they perceived. What they have shared may or may not be the whole story. The facility may have a very different take on the situation, which they cannot share with you. In my professional career as an advocate, I have often found that families often have unrealistic expectations of facilities and blame the facility for not providing the care they want for their loved ones. Remember, long-term care facilities do **NOT** provide one-on-one care for residents.

If your loved one is in the hospital due to a crisis, do not let the social worker or case manager force you to move your loved one because they are in a hurry to discharge them. You will need the time to talk with the facility and tour the home before you know if it is a good fit for your loved one.

Do not wait for a crisis to do your planning. Anyone eighteen and older should have powers of attorney in place. If you are married or have children, you need to have a plan to honor your wishes in case of a crisis. The time to do this is before a crisis. If you wait for the crisis, it may be too late. You must be cognitively able to make your wishes known to draw up the documents. (Depending on the State you live in, a wife or child may **be unable** to make decisions for you when you cannot make them yourself.) Your goal and the purpose of this book is to help you become proactive, not reactive.

Don't expect a long-term facility to correct a lifetime of problems with a loved one! I have seen families who make complaints about a facility because their loved one is not getting a bath. Upon investigating the issue, I found out that this individual always had an issue with bathing. Before moving them in, the family knew about the issue and expected the long-term care facility to correct it. Not only is that wrong, but that is not fair to do the your loved one or the staff of the facility! Residents have a right to refuse any care, and the facility cannot force them to do something they do not want to do. I have also seen this same principle with residents who are chronic complainers, those who may be sexually inappropriate, residents who are racist, or bullies. Understand when you move a loved one into a long-term care facility, it is not their job to correct a lifetime of bad behaviors.

Families need to understand that long-term care facilities do not provide one-on-one care. A long-term care facility is an institutional setting and follows State and/or Federal laws that govern the care provided to each resident. You need to be sure your expectations of care are reasonable and not something that could only be provided in a one-on-one situation.

Example 18: Example Of An Unreasonable Expectation

> *I had a Director of Nursing call me, requesting I handle a situation where the staff refused to help a resident put on her makeup in the morning. This seemed like a normal request until I asked the staff why. It turns out that this particular woman's makeup routine was approximately three hours long, and according to the resident and her family, nothing could be skipped. In the ensuing conversation with the family and the resident, I explained that while she certainly had the right to have her makeup done a certain way, it would be unrealistic to expect a community to provide a staff member to assist her every day with a three-hour makeup routine.*

This family's expectation of what a long-term care facility can do was unreasonable.

Do not let any well-meaning friend or family member try and tell you that you should not move your loved one in a long-term care facility; you should continue to care for them at home. It is easy for someone on the outside to say that, but they are not the ones giving up their lives, sometimes at a great personal loss. Their families, jobs, or health are not suffering because the burden of care is falling on you, not them. You will know when it is time to place a loved one. Remember, you will be no good for anyone unless you care for yourself first. Sometimes, the most loving thing you can do for a loved one is place them in the best facility possible and then become an advocate for their needs.

Once you place your loved one in their new home, I highly recommend you get a copy of my first book, I *Am The Resident – Becoming The Advocate For Your Loved One's Needs*. This book explains all the federal resident rights in terms families can understand and includes 64 examples of how I used these rights to get my residents the care they wanted when their facility told them they were not required to honor their requests. The book can be ordered on Amazon or on my website, advocacy4seniors.com.

Chapter 16

I've Made My Decision. What Happens Next?

Now that you have chosen, let the facility know your intent to apply for placement. It is important for families to understand that just because you have chosen the facility does NOT mean that the one you selected will accept your loved one. Under federal law, a facility does not have to accept everyone who applies. You may be wondering why a facility would refuse the acceptance of a resident. There could be many reasons, including but not limited to.

- They do not feel they could meet your loved one's needs.

    a. If your loved one has dementia, the staff at the facility you have selected may not be trained in how to care for residents with dementia.

    b. Some facilities do not accept younger residents; they specialize in the geriatric population.

    c. They may not be trained to care for those with mental illness or developmental disabilities.

    d. Sometimes, they have so many residents who require a high level of care that they cannot accept more residents with high care needs due to not having enough staff to meet the needs of the residents.

e. You may not require the level of care the provided.

It is important to understand that they may say no and do not have to explain why your loved one is not being accepted. This is why you always want to have another choice ready when you are going through the process.

Example 19: Respect The Process, or Your Loved One Will Lose

I was working with a family, assisting them in finding a skilled nursing home for their mom. The daughter was very impatient with the staff at the different facilities she toured. She told them / demanded that if her mom came to their facility, she would expect them to follow all her instructions. When the facility met her mom, the staff reported that she was a sweet woman and seemed easy to get along with. However, the daughter constantly called the admissions person and tried to push them to rush their decision. In the end, the facility denied the woman's move to their facility. The facility does not have to explain why they do not accept someone. When I called and spoke with the social worker, she told me that they did not feel they could meet the resident's needs. I was left wondering if the real reason was that the facility did not want to deal with the daughter and all her demands.

- If your loved one is in the hospital, you can contact their social worker or case manager and request that their records be sent over.

- If your loved one is being transferred from another facility, call the facility, and let them know you want the records sent over. It will help to give them the name and fax number of the person you want the records sent to. The long-term care community will want to see the following when deciding if they can meet the needs of your loved one.

  a. The history and physical.

  b. Medication list.

  c. Doctor's orders and progress notes.

  d. The nurse notes.

  e. Social Service notes.

  f. A copy of the face sheet.

- If your loved one is living on their own or with you, they will need you to contact their doctor and have the records faxed over. The doctor's office should know what to send, but generally, they will want.

a.   The medical history
b.   Medication list
c.   Notes from the most current visit
d.   Recent hospitalization notes.

Once the records are received, the nursing staff will review the records and see if the placement is appropriate. This process usually takes a few days to complete from the time the medical records are received.

If your loved one is accepted, congratulations, you are ready to proceed and arrange transportation. If they are not, go to your second choice and request that their records be sent over to them for review.

Once you have chosen a facility that best meets the needs of your loved one, what happens next? Hopefully, your loved one has been actively involved in the selection process, but what if that was not possible and your loved one says they do not want to go into a long-term care facility? This can be a very difficult/ stressful time as you decide how to let your loved one know that you can no longer care for them at home or that they are no longer able to live alone. *Note: The most important thing to remember in this situation is that you cannot force your loved one to move into a long-term care facility. Under State and Federal laws, they have a right to refuse. Knowing this, you will have to come up with a plan to help them come to the understanding that they need to move.* Here are some tips on how you can approach this topic.

- Try talking to your loved one and explaining why they must be placed. Sometimes, making it about yourself can make all the difference. Say something like I need to know that you are in a safe place. I worry so much about you that I am starting to have issues myself. Or you can say, "Mom, I can no longer care for you; I don't feel qualified to provide all the care you need."

- You can ask their doctor to write an order for your loved one stating that he/she feels like they need to be in a long-term care facility.

- Sometimes, suggesting that they go to a facility for a month so you can get some much-needed respite (rest) may work. Often, seniors have heard so many negative stories about facilities that they can't imagine any facility would be a good move. You have done all the research and found a facility that can meet their needs. Many facilities do allow respite stays (short-term stays.) If your loved one goes in for respite, they may find out it is not as bad as they imagined. I have done this many times and had the residents reach out to their children and ask if they could stay.

- If your loved one is unwilling to make the move, you may need to make an appointment with their doctor and have them evaluated to see if maybe there has been a change in their ability to make sound medical decisions.

Now that you have found placement for your loved one take a deep breath and know that you have done everything you can to ensure your loved one is placed in a facility that best meets their needs.

Congratulations! Your role now will change from being the caregiver to becoming an advocate for your loved one!

—————— *Chapter 17* ——————

Epilogue

Placing a loved one in a long-term care facility can be very traumatic for both your loved one and yourself. Realize that this is not going to be an easy journey, and give yourself time to grieve and adjust to your loved one's new living situation. While finding the best placement for your loved one, don't neglect to care for yourself and your family. You cannot be a good advocate for your loved one if you get sick.

If you have ever been on an airplane, you will see the flight attendants give you directions in case of an emergency. They will always say that if oxygen masks are deployed, put yours on first and then place the mask on your children. This is because if you are not taken care of, you will not be able to care for your children. The same is true when being a caregiver for your loved ones. Just because you are moving them to a long-term care community does not mean you will not be caring for them. However, your role will change. Instead of being the direct caregiver for your loved one, you have moved them to a facility that is better qualified to provide the care they need, giving them the ability to achieve the highest quality of life possible. You have now gone from being the direct caregiver to being the advocate for your loved one. No one is more qualified to advocate for your loved one than you. I am a professional case manager/advocate for seniors, but I always refer to the resident or their families because you know your loved ones better than I ever will. You have the history that often unlocks the keys to resolving the issues your loved one faces.

Example 20: Knowing The Person's History Can Unlock The Mystery.

I had a skilled nursing home resident in a memory care unit who tried to elope every day at 2 p.m. (walk away) from the facility. The nursing home contacted me and said they were going to have to send a discharge notice to the resident if I could not figure out why he was trying to leave. I met with the staff and the resident and asked the staff what this man's job was. They did not know. I asked them to contact his family and ask them that question. The staff got back to me and told me they spoke with the family and found out that this man was a used car salesman, so that did not explain why he was trying to walk away every day at 2 p.m. I then asked them to contact the family again and ask if they could contact anyone he worked with and ask them if there was something this man did every day

*at 2 p.m. We found out that every day at 2 p.m., it
was this man's job to check the lot!*

This man was not trying to leave the nursing home; he was doing his job! I had the staff call the family again to find his co-workers' names. From that day forward, every day at 1:45 p.m., the staff went up to this man and told him he did not need to check the lot; John (name of a co-worker) was going to check the lot for him that day. The man stopped trying to leave the facility. He never tried to leave the nursing home; he was doing his job. Without the insight from the family, we could never have resolved this issue.

Families are the most important part of the team when a resident has dementia or any cognitive deficiency and cannot communicate their needs!

Definitions

Assisted Living Facilities (ALF) – Part of the continuum of care that provides a combination of housing and personal care services and health care designed to respond to individuals who need assistance with normal daily activities in a way that promotes maximum independence.

Centers for Medicare & Medicaid Services (CMS): A federal agency that plays a key role in the overall direction of the healthcare system. CMS is responsible for regulating and paying nursing homes, home health agencies, and hospices for the care of Medicare and Medicaid (in conjunction with the states) beneficiaries.

Dementia: A general term for loss of memory and other mental abilities severe enough to interfere with daily life. Structural and physiological changes in the brain cause it. Alzheimer's disease is the most common type of dementia. Among those ages 70 and older living in nursing homes in 2019, 70% had dementia.

Department of Health & Senior Services (DHSS): The Department of Health and Senior Services is responsible for managing and promoting all public health programs to improve life and wellness for Missourians. They are responsible for maintaining programs to control and prevent disease, regulation, and licensure of health, and programs designed to create safeguards and health resources for seniors and the state's vulnerable populations. DHSS is the agency that monitors long-term care facilities and operates the Elder Abuse & Neglect Hotline.

Elder Abuse & Neglect Hotline: The hotline is operated by the staff of the Department of Health & Senior Services. A report can be made online (health.mo.gov › safety › abuse) or by calling 800.392.0210 and filing a report over the phone.

Intermediate Care Facility (ICF): The facility provides 24-hour accommodation, board, personal care, and basic health and nursing care services under the daily supervision of a licensed nurse and the direction of a licensed physician to three or more residents dependent for care and supervision. A licensed Nursing Home Administrator is required.

Long-Term Care Ombudsman: Ombudsman are the federally mandated advocates for residents in long-term care facilities. Ombudsmen are the experts in both Federal and State Laws that govern the long-term care facilities of each State. The ombudsman can advocate for any resident in long-term care and work with the facilities to ensure the resident's rights are honored. The ombudsman always tries and resolve issues to the satisfaction of the resident. At the end of each day, the family, staff, and advocates go home, and the resident remains in the facility. This is their home, and we all want our wishes honored in our homes! The Long-Term Care Ombudsman services are free to all residents and their families.

Medicaid: The federal and state-approved, state-operated public assistance program that pays for healthcare services to low-income people, including older adults or disabled persons who qualify. Medicaid pays for long-term nursing home care and some limited home health services, and it may pay for some assisted living services depending on the state. It is the largest public payer of long-term care services, especially nursing home care. Each state can determine the extent of what services it will cover above a certain federally required minimum.

Medicare: The federal program that provides medical insurance for people aged 65 and older, some disabled persons, and those with end-stage renal disease. It provides physician, hospital, and medical benefits for individuals over 65 or those meeting specific disability standards. Benefits for nursing home and home health services are limited to short-term rehabilitative care. Different parts of Medicare cover specific services if you meet certain conditions.

Pathway To Safety: Pathway to safety states that a resident in a residential care facility or assisted living facility must be able to get out of the building in an emergency with minimal assistance in five minutes or less.

Preadmission Screening and Resident Review – PASRR: This is the federal requirement to help ensure that individuals with mental illness, intellectual disabilities, or related conditions are not inappropriately placed in a nursing facility for long-term care.

Residential Care Facility: Residential care facility means any residence, other than an ALF, intermediate care facility, or skilled nursing facility, which provides 24-hour care to three or more adults who need or are provided with shelter, board, and protective oversight, which may include storage and distribution or administration of medications and care during short term illness or recuperation.

Skilled Nursing Facility (SNF): A residential care setting that provides 24-hour care to individuals who are chronically ill or disabled. Individuals must be unable to care for themselves.

Transfer of Assets: Missouri HealthNet has a five-year look-back period when an individual applies for Medicaid. A transfer of assets that would incur a penalty occurs when someone transfers those assets out of a person's name five years prior to entering a nursing home.

Resources

Alzheimer's Association

Website: alz.org

24/7 Helpline: 800.272.3900

Center for Medicare & Medicaid Services (CMS)

Website: cms.gov

Consumer Voice - theconsumervoice.org

Consumer Voice is the leading national voice representing consumers in issues related to long-term care, helping to ensure that consumers are empowered to advocate for themselves. They are a primary source of information and tools for consumers, families, caregivers, advocates, and Ombudsmen to help ensure quality care for the individual.

TheConsumerVoice.org/get help - This website will get you to a page where you can see a map of the State's Long-term care Ombudsman programs.

Department of Health & Senior Services (DHSS): DHSS is the regulatory agency in Missouri.

Website: health.mo.gov

Elder Abuse & Neglect Hotline: The hotline is operated by the staff of the Department of Health & Senior Services. A report can be made online (https://apps4.mo.gov/APS_Portal) or by calling 800.392.0210 and filing a report over the phone.

Long-Term Care Ombudsman Program
Website: Missouri-health.mo.gov/seniors/ombudsman

Long-Term Care Ombudsman Regions In Missouri

Young at Heart Resources
1304 N. Walnut, Suite 150,
Cameron, MO 64429
(660) 240-9400
Fax: (816) 396-0568
www.yahresources.org/

VOYCE
8050 Watson Road
St. Louis, MO 63119
(314) 918-8222 or
(866) 918-8222
http://www.voycestl.org/

Mid-America Regional Council
600 Broadway, Suite 200
Kansas City, MO 64105-1536
(816) 474-4240
Fax: (816) 421-7758
www.marc.org/

Care Connection for Aging Services
106 W. Young St
Warrensburg, MO 64093
(660) 747-3107 or (800) 748-7826
Fax: (660) 747-3100
www.goaging.org/

Aging Best
201 W. Broadway, Bldg. 1 – Suite E
Columbia, MO 65203
(573) 443-5823 or (800) 369-5211
Fax: (573) 875-8907
www.agingbest.org/

Aging Matters
1078 Wolverine, Suite J
Cape Girardeau, MO 63701
(573) 335-3331 or (800) 392-8771
Fax: (573) 335-3017
www.agingmatters2u.com/

Council of Churches of the Ozarks
3055 E. Division St.
Springfield, MO 65802
(417) 862-3598
Fax: (417) 862-2129
www.ccozarks.org

MO HealthNet, a/k/a Missouri Medicaid

Website: https://dss.mo.gov/mhd/

National Academy of Elder Law Attorneys (NAELA)

Website: naela.org

Nursing Home Compare

https://www.medicare.gov/care-compare/?providerType=Nurs
ingHome

Show Me Long Term Care in Missouri (use this website to view complaints/inspection reports.

Website: https://healthapps.dhss.mo.gov/showmeltc/default.
aspx

I Am The Resident – Becoming An Advocate For Your Loved One's Needs (Available on Amazon in eBook or print, ordered through your local bookstore, or can be ordered through the publisher BookBaby at https://store.bookbaby.com/book/I-am-the-Resident, or directly from my website advocacy4seniors.com)

Overview

I Am The Resident – Becoming An Advocate For Your Loved One's Needs is written to teach families, students, and professionals how to advocate for loved ones/clients in long-term care communities. This book takes the Federal Regulations as they pertain to resident rights and explains them in simple, easy-to-understand terms that can help individuals resolve problems in a long-term care community when they arise. The book includes 64 real-life examples of advocacy in action. This is a great resource for any family who has placed a loved one in a long-term care community and wants to ensure that their loved one receives the highest level of care.

Author: Cheryl J. Wilson, M.S.

Website: advocavy4seniors.com

Check this website often for updates on long-term care issues, ask questions, request a private consultation, or book a speaking engagement.

Appendix 1

Pros & Cons Checklist

Name of Facility:

Address:

Phone Number:

Date of Visit:

Pros	Cons

Notes:

Appendix 2

Placement Checklist

Name of Facility:

Address:

Phone Number:

Date of Visit:

	Yes	No	Notes
General Questions			
Is it necessary to place your loved one? (Is your loved one safe where they are now?)			
Do you know the level of care needed? Residential/Assisted Living/ Intermediate or Skilled Care.)			
Will you need a Medicaid Bed?			
Have you completed your online research on Medicare.gov?			
Does the facility's inspection report show quality-of-care problems?			
Has the facility corrected all deficiencies?			
Has the facility been cited for abuse issues in the last few years?			

Is there information on how to file a grievance?			
How and when are families notified of changes in the resident's physical and mental condition?			
Do they offer transportation? Is transportation Medicaid-approved? (Some facilities only provide transportation at a private pay rate and are not contracted with a transportation company that is a Medicaid provider)			
Do you know all the charges and fees?			
Are there extra charges for services such as beauty shop, personal phone, television, and internet?			
Get copies of everything you sign and all the admission paperwork.			
Does the facility use agency staff?			
Do you have the admissions person's contact information?			
Touring A Facility – Environment			
Did you notice any unpleasant odors?			
Is the temperature comfortable for the residents?			
Is the lighting good for the residents?			
Is the noise level comfortable?			
Is the furniture in good repair?			
Are the exits marked clearly?			

Are handrails and grab bars appropriately placed in bathrooms and hallways?			
Residents			
Were the residents clean, and well-groomed?			
Are residents in restraints?			
Are the residents engaged with each other?			
Are the residents sitting around the nurse's station, or are they engaged with each other?			
Dinning & Food			
Are there flexible mealtimes?			
Do residents have a choice of food items at each meal?			
Can the facility provide special diets?			
Are snacks available?			
Are staff available to help residents eat when needed?			
Staff			
Do staff knock before entering a room?			
Do staff refer to residents by their preferred names?			
Did the staff's relationship with residents appear to be respectful?			
What is the resident-to-staff ratio?			
What is the turnover rate for the administrative staff and direct caregivers?			

Is there a social service staff available to me?			
Residents' Room			
Can residents have personal belongings and furniture in my room?			
Do residents have a closet and drawers for my belongings?			
Do residents have access to the internet, a computer, a personal phone, and television?			
Activities			
Is there a variety of activities offered?			
Are activities offered seven days a week during the day and evening?			
Do residents have input into the activities?			
Do the residents seem to enjoy the activities?			
Are outdoor and out trips available for residents?			
Are staff available to help residents go outside?			
Does the facility have a family council?			
Does the facility have volunteers?			
Does the facility have an Ombudsman?			
Does the facility offer the religious or cultural support I need?			
Residents with Dementia			

Does the facility have a Secure Special Care Unit?			
Have you seen the Disclosure Statement?			
What if any dementia training is provided for staff?			
What is the percentage of residents with dementia?			
What is your approach to dementia care?			
How are activities in the special care unit different than activities in the general population?			
How do you work with challenging behaviors?			
Do the residents have room to wander indoors? Outdoors, such as an enclosed courtyard?			

About the Author

I have been a Geriatric Care Manager for over 27 years. I specialize in issues surrounding long-term care communities and the unique needs of residents with dementia. I have worked in long-term care facilities as a Certified Nurse's Aide and Certified Medical Technician; I have had family members in long-term care and was the Director of Ombudsman Services and Lead Advocate for the St. Louis Long-Term Care Ombudsman Program for over 17 years. With experience working, having loved ones in a long-term community, and having 27 years as an advocate for residents in long-term care, I believe I am uniquely qualified to help the residents, staff, and families come together to resolve situations that can arise in the long-term care communities. I have a master's degree in Gerontology and had the pleasure of doing my practicum study with the St. Louis Alzheimer's Association, where I came into direct contact with families struggling with care for loved ones with dementia in their homes as well as those who had loved ones in long-term care communities. During my time with the Alzheimer's Association, I saw the need for individuals who specialized in advocating for individuals with dementia. Over the years, I have seen many things, but one thing I know needs to happen is that family members need to have access to the regulations and understand resident rights before problems arise.

When conflicts arise, it is often because the resident was moved to a long-term care facility that they should have never been admitted to. Long-term care facilities, like any other business, specialize in different areas. Families need to know how to find a facility that can best meet the needs of their loved ones.

A Complete Guide To Moving A Loved One In A Long-Term Care Facility was written to walk a family through the process of finding a long-term care facility that can best meet the needs of their loved ones. When a resident is properly placed, they will be in a facility where they can achieve the quality of life they're looking for and give you the peace of mind of knowing that your loved one is in a safe, caring environment.

Cheryl J. Wilson, M.S.

Printed in the United States
by Baker & Taylor Publisher Services